Passion for Healing and Wellbeing

Second Edition

This book is dedicated to my Grandmother, Wilhelmina Sufragan, who fought breast cancer yet survived to live a healthy life for twenty more years. She was a remarkable woman.

And to my Mom, Wanda Marchewka, who from the very first day believed in my chosen method of healing, and who still prepares delicious dishes out of raw vegetables for me.

Other book written by Alexandra Zawieracz

"Passion for Healthy Foods"
Alex's Food Choices

Passion for Healing and Wellbeing

Alex's Breast Cancer Story

Alexandra Zawieracz

"Some men see things as they are and ask why.
Others dream things that never were and ask why not."
George Bernard Shaw

"The world can only change from within"
Eckhart Tolle

Why am I writing my story?

Once I was diagnosed with cancer I was overwhelmed with the urge to find out everything about it and to explore all available choices. I knew only to some degree I could rely on doctors. None of my friends or relatives had the knowledge or experience in fighting cancer. It was all up to me. I had to understand every aspect of my new life; I needed to know what path to take, physically and emotionally, in order to become cancer free. I have started the process of reading many books, researching, browsing the internet and found myself overwhelmed with the information available. Each day I was learning something very important and each day I was forgetting some of the important lessons from the day before. It occurred to me that the only way to retain the knowledge was to start writing down the essence of everything I wanted to remember and to apply to my life. This is how this book has started.

Life is beautiful, especially when we realize the potential of it.

Author's contact information:
azawieracz@austin.rr.com
http://www.alexandrazawieracz.com,

Table of Contents

March 4	Where to look for alkaline water How safe is fluoride
March 7	Why multivitamins and minerals are important Difference between synthetic and natural vitamins - How to read labels
March 9	Buckwheat (Kasha) & Quinoa
March 11	Root canal teeth - tooth extraction Mercury and Calcium Bentonite Clay
March 13	Second breast surgery
March 16	Food combining Ice-cold foods or beverages
March 19	Second surgery biopsy results
March 26	Appointment with oncologist. Tamoxifen
March 27	Colon hydrotherapy appointment
March 28	Ways to Think Our Way Into Good Health
March 30	Gas and bloating and Solution
April 1	Budwig Protocol – Flaxseed oil and cheese
April 4	Farmer's Markets
April 7	Build self confidence
April 8	How our thoughts can cause or cure cancer, or any other illness
April 9	How the body works
April 10	Understanding Health

February 2

The Beginning
Cancer Healing Facts

I read that writing down our thoughts brings peace to the mind. I also read that when diagnosed with cancer, it helps to keep track of everything connected to remember and understand the process of healing. This is one of the reasons I have decided to write about my journey, which is also an inexpensive way to give myself therapy.

Once I discovered a lump in my right breast, I went through several tests, including a diagnostic mammogram, ultrasound, biopsy, and PEM scan and on January 14 I was diagnosed with the breast cancer. All tests proved that I have a malignant tumor. I believe that in the end I will be fine; however, I need to change some of my habits and learn more about a healthy preventive lifestyle. I know that I truly can take responsibility for my own health and change my condition. I am spending hours on research through the internet and many books; this is one fight I don't want to lose. I have already learned important facts. I intend to get all the information to understand my choices, make right decisions and become healthier than ever. Today is the beginning. The following days provide more detail regarding each point listed below.

1. Take high doses of CoQ10, 300 – 400 mg of gel form, along with a complete balanced antioxidant and mineral.
2. The immune system needs 9–10 hours of sleep in total darkness to recharge completely.
3. The cause of cancer is low cellular oxygenation levels. Increasing oxygen levels kills cancerous cells. Eating alkaline versus acidic foods increases level of oxygen. Alkalinizing the body is one of the basic strategies in the battle against cancer, and in improving our health in general.
4. Flaxseed oil added to cottage cheese is a well known cancer treatment, it is called Budwig Protocol. It provides essential fatty acids needed by cell walls so that oxygen can enter the cells.
5. Some doctors believe that cancer is a fungus disease. One strategy is to attack cancer by alkalinizing the

digestive track. Patients drink three teaspoons a day of baking soda with water 30 minutes before breakfast.

6. Colon cleaning needs to happen on the journey to good health, use fiber.
7. There is a correlation between low enzyme levels and cancer. Pancreatic enzymes destroy cancer cells.
8. Expose yourself to sun at least 20 minutes a day, no sunscreen. Or take supplemental D.
9. Do not use microwave.
10. Remove any root canal teeth, every one of them has huge amounts of toxins.
11. Drink good water, Alkaline water if possible, and lots of it!
12. Exercise regularly.
13. Develop "Peace of Mind". "I lovingly forgive and release all of the past. I choose to fill my world with joy. I love and approve of myself".
14. Eliminate excessive intake of proteins and fats, processed and cooked foods, refined sugars, oils and carbohydrates. Eat more vegetables and fruits.
15. Eat organic whenever possible.
16. Eliminate environmental toxins to give your body a fighting chance.
17. ELIMINATE SUGAR – IT FEEDS CANCER.

February 3

Cancer Diagnose
Why Natural Ways of Healing

Today I had the PEM scan follow up appointment with my surgeon, Dr. Jane. The scan confirmed presence of a malignant cancer. The good news is that the cancer is located only in the tumor; the rest of the breast is free. I came to my appointment with a list of questions: how much CoQ10 to take, does Rice Bran Extract kill cancerous cells, will Melatonin help me not just sleep but fight the cancer, and more. She knew nothing about any of these remedies, her world is limited to surgeries only, and surgery is what we decided to do. The lumpectomy is scheduled for February 17, Tuesday. On Monday they will do all necessary tests to prepare me for the next day. I took a week off from work for recovery.

To be honest, I do not think the surgery is required. The natural treatments that I am learning about eliminate tumors and cancer. However, I need more information to stop blindly follow doctor's recommendations, and be aware of risks that I might take. I am starting to believe in natural ways of healing, and will try them to eliminate chemo, radiation, and taking Tamoxifen that destroy not only cancerous cells, but my healthy cells as well.

I believe there are three main reasons people die of cancer today are:
> 1) Lack of information
> 2) Lack of discipline once they have the information
> 3) Blind trust in cancer doctors

Unfortunately no natural substance can be advertised as a cure for cancer, this is Federal law. My research proved that cancer is one of the most profitable businesses in the USA; millions of dollars are made from selling prescription drugs, recommending natural ways of healing does not support the drug business and represents serious competition to what MDs stand for. Ironically drugs are the third reason why people die, the first two are cancer and heart failure. Doctors put themselves or their clinics/hospitals at legal and professional risk unless they use radiation, surgery and drugs. The cutting-edge cancer clinics in the world are located outside of the United States. The practice of curing cancer , a common outcome in alternative cancer clinics, has been outlawed in the United States. It is actually illegal for a master herbalist, for example, to even attempt to cure a patient of cancer. Much of what is considered as alternative in our country is part of the conventional standard of care in Europe and Asia, where alternative therapies have been helping people for centuries

When women in America have breast cancer and go to see their oncologists, they are not told about the link between healthy diet and halting the spread of cancer. They are also not told how they can stop the spread of their cancers by taking supplements.

Fact: Most drugs treat the symptoms, but not the underlying problem.

February 6

Treatment Strategy

I am continuing my research. I learned that chemotherapy and radiation are used because cancer cells are weaker than normal cells and therefore may die first. However, chemo and radiation damage respiratory enzymes in healthy cells, and overload them with toxins, so they become more likely to develop into cancer. The cancer conditions are worsened, not improved. And the cancer usually returns a second time unless changes are made to support the healthy body, such as diet, exercise, and a stress free life. Submitting to conventional chemo treatments for breast cancer makes a woman a patient for life due to all the organ problems likely to occur as a result of the chemo.

I feel I have enough information to decide on my treatment strategy. I can not loose any more time, I have to start the recovery now. I chose the cancer treatment described by Bill Henderson, I have to follow his regiment diligently and I will be cancer free. Yep, this is true!

Below is the summary of what I will do for the following months. The cancer diet starts now. I will start using cancer killing products as soon as they arrive; I placed them on order today. All this will restore my body's balance and remove cancer cells.

Daily intake:

1. **Beta Glucan**
   Immune system stimulator, for production of white blood cells, cellular mobilization, phagocytic capacity, production of oxygen.
   In the morning (1,000 mg), 30 minutes before eating or drinking anything. See April 11.

2. **Cottage Cheese / Flaxseed Oil (The Budwig Protocol)**
   Provides essential fatty acids needed by cell walls so that oxygen can enter the cells
   2/3 cup of organic, low fat cottage cheese with 4-6 tablespoons of oil. I add pineapple with stevia or organic berries for flavor. See April 1.

3. **Heart Plus and Green Tea Extract**
   Digestion, mood maintenance, immune enchantment, detoxification and energy enchancement.
   Heart Plus includes Rose Hips, Lysine, Proline and Green Tea Extract (3,600 mg). Take together with food or between meals, does not matter.

4. **Barley Power**
   Builds alkaline system and is nature's complete concentration of nutrition for maintaining health.
   15 minutes before each meal, or 2 hours after eating if having 2 meals only. 6,120 mg

5. **Amazon Herbs**
   Support immune system and healthy cell division, prevent abnormal cell growth, stimulate circulatory and lymphatic functions.
   Gravizon with Graviola
   Cat's Claw, bark of Una de Gato
   Fibrezon, fiber for internal cleansing program

6. **Cancer Diet**
   Very efficient and thorough cleanse of the entire digestive system and perverts cancer.

   I avoid sugar, processed and cooked food, avoid acidic foods, animal protein, dairy, and gluten. I maximize the raw vegetables and gluten-free bread products, lentils, seeds, and nuts but no peanuts. The most powerful cancer-fighting vegetables are: broccoli, cabbage, brussel sprouts, mustard greens, kale, cauliflower, beet, ginger, onion, garlic, mint, parsley, avocados, tomatoes, carrots, celery, cilantro, parsnips, peppers, beets, and mushrooms.

7. Vitamins / Mineral Supplements

Multi-nutrient formula as directed
BiOmega3: 3,000 mg
CoQ10: 300 mg; produces energy in cells (see June 5)
Vitamin E: 1,000 IU; enhances immunity
Vitamin C: 6,000 mg; antioxidant that gets rid of free radicals
Vitamin D: see September 19
Wobenzymes: 3,600; 30 minutes before each meal; they are metabolic enzymes supporting immune system and all body functions
Digestive enzymes, with each meal
Probiotics

This program works because it addresses the four characteristics of cancer:

- brings more oxygen to the cells
- helps the body change from acidic to alkaline
- detoxifies the body
- boosts the immune system

Something to remember: supplements should complement our healthy diet, not serve as a replacement. There's simply no substitute for eating healthy unprocessed whole foods.

See April 11 for my treatment update.

February 11

Cancer Test

Today I sent urine sample for cancer testing, it went all the way to Philippines. This test looks at abnormally dividing cells and tells the relative number or level of these cells. The test returns a single number. If that number is 50 or more there is cancer that requires treatment. If the number is zero to 49, there is no cancer. The reading should come in a week. I will repeat this test 6-8 weeks from now. If there is no progress I will consider other alternatives.

The Barley Power, Beta Glucan and other products arrived. I am currently taking 94 tablets a day, 3 different times a day. Wow, I never thought I'd be swallowing so much; well, better to take herbs than chemicals.

February 13

Eating Right

I have realized that the moment I was diagnosed with cancer I became a survivor. People say that everything happens for a reason, I believe this is true. The reason why I have cancer is because it is time to change my life; the way I think, eat, take care of myself, appreciate what I have and what every day offers me. This is the time to meet myself and begin knowing who I am meant to be. I am also learning to honor myself by saying no to things I don't want to do and letting go of things I cannot change.

For two weeks now I have been on the 'cancer' diet, it is not like a macrobiotic diet, it is more strict and does not allow cooked or processed food. It is not about reducing sugar, saturated fat, animal protein and dairy; it is about removing all of it and eating only whole vegetables, sprouted and preservative free breads, fruit, seeds and nuts. Every morning I eat organic cottage cheese with flaxseed oil, and I love it. Once cottage cheese is well mixed with flaxseed oil it looses its dairy characteristics. Each day I add different fruit; yesterday I had it with black berries, today with a fresh pineapple. It tastes great! I think everyone should have this breakfast; people would be healthier.

Every day I eat servings of fruits and vegetables, they reduce breast cancer recurrence by 40%. Scientists from the University of California examined the relationship between plasma carotenoid concentration in fruit and vegetable and their intake in 1,550 women previously treated for early stage breast cancer. After 5 years of follow-up, those women with the highest plasma carotenoid concentrations had a 40% reduced risk for breast cancer recurrence. (*Journal of Clinical Oncology*, September, 2005).

Carotenoids are natural fat-soluble colorful pigments found in carrots, spinach, kale, cantaloupe, tomatoes, pink grapefruit, watermelon, papaya, apricots, dark green leafy vegetables and blueberries.

Salads full of these colorful vegetables should always be eaten with some type of fat. The moderate use of extra virgin olive oil or avocado in a salad significantly enhanced the absorption of all carotenoids (alpha-carotene, beta-carotene, lycopene, and lutein.

Fruits and nuts are another tasty combination. The healthy fats found in the nuts will bring to life all the carotenoids in the fruits. Snacking on dried fruits and nuts satisfies the sweet tooth while loading up the body with carotenoids. For best digestion, eat the fruits first and then the nuts rather than eating them together.

When considering nuts eliminate peanuts. Peanuts are especially problematic, as they have no omega-3 and therefore distort your omega 6:3 ratio. They are also frequently contaminated with a carcinogenic mold called aflatoxin, and are one of the most pesticide-contaminated crops.

Almost all fruits and vegetables have anti-cancer activity. The superstars of the research labs are garlic and onions, broccoli, cabbage, kale, mushrooms, Brussels sprouts, greens, carrots, celery, cilantro, parsley, parsnips, tomatoes, peppers, flax seeds, citrus, and soy. However, soy should not be eaten unless it is fermented in the traditional oriental manner and eaten as a small part of a mineral and protein rich meal.

I created my own cook book filled with delicious recipes, it is called "Passion for Healthy Foods". They all are very healthy and delicious. I had no idea how tasty kale can be, how many healthy options there are for salad dressing, things we can do with beans that I never considered, etc. Yesterday I made sundried tomato hummus, it was better than others I have purchased; and my sprouted green lentils salad is amazing.

Fact: Vegetables to avoid: corn and iceberg lettuce. Corn is a tender plant, and is heavily sprayed - on the average of every 10 days, and often every 4 to 5 days. Corn, like cotton, is subject to many plant diseases, as well as many insect pests. In addition, it is generally grown on bare ground, in order to prevent competition for nutrients by weeds. For this reason, the ground is also drenched with herbicides - beginning before it is seeded. Head lettuce, or "iceberg" lettuce is also a very tender plant, and also suffers from many diseases and insect pests. For these reasons all head and iceberg lettuce crops are heavily and often sprayed.

February 16

On The Way to Hospital

This morning I went to St. David's hospital for pre-surgery testing; blood, urine and chest x-rays. On the way there I crashed into another car. We were at an intersection, the car in front of me moved, I moved too and while looking to the left I did not notice that the car stopped. The damage was small, however, big enough for my insurance to be involved. Instead of doing an insurance claim the man said that his car is old and he can live with the scratches, he said that he likes to work on cars and will replace the light himself. He asked that I only pay for the part. He took my phone number and said he will call me with the cost. Moral: there are good people around us, I am lucky to have many of them in my life.

February 18

Breast Surgery

Yesterday morning I arrived in the hospital at 6:10am for the 8:00am surgery. My family and friends were with me before the surgery and after. Once the surgery was over, Dr. Jane came out to the waiting room to announce the results. She said that the tumor came out easily, was small, and only required a small incision to be removed. She was able to do it low on the breast even though the tumor was high to conceal my scar. She took one lymph node for testing. She said that she has to wait for the lab results to see what kind of cancer and how

19

aggressive it is to decide what treatment to recommend. She will discuss this with me once the results come back, at my appointment next week. When I saw her before the surgery, she said that the x-rays from the day before showed a spot on my lung. The CAT scan of my chest is scheduled for Friday. When I see Dr. Jane next week she'll have the results. I am sure it will be nothing.

On a funny note, when I came back from the anesthesia, nurse told me that the first thing I said out loud was 'Love wins', of course I do not remember it but all nurses thought it was hilarious.

During the last two days I received beautiful flowers, phone calls, and emails with positive energy. It feels good to know how many people care about me.

February 19

Biopsy Results

Dr. Jane called me just after 5:00pm, the tumor and lymph node biopsy results came back. The lymph node test is negative, cancer did not spread. However, the cancer in the tumor is invasive and tumor's margins were not clear. I need additional surgery; more breast tissue has to be removed to make sure that there are no cancerous cells left.

First I felt disappointed; this is not what I wanted to hear. Later I have realized that this is actually good news; the cancer did not spread, whatever is left in the breast will be removed soon, and I will continue my journey to the full recovery.

February 20

Processed and Cooked Foods (DEAD foods)

Going back to my research; when I talk about eliminating processed and cooked foods as part of the cancer diet regime, I am being asked what these foods are. Here is good explanation.

Traditional **food processing** had two functions: to make food more digestible and to preserve it. In the past, processing was carried out by farmers and artisans such as bread makers, cheese makers, distillers, millers and so forth. This type of processing resulted in delicious foods. The traditional processing enhances the nutrient value of our foods. Traditional bread making neutralizes anti-nutrients in grains to make the minerals more available; lacto-fermentation of cabbage to make sauerkraut increases the levels of vitamin C and many B vitamin; and the making of yogurt, kefir and similar products from fresh milk makes the nutrients in the milk more available and more digestible. Unfortunately, in modern times we have abandoned local artesian processing in favor of factory and industrial processing, which destroys the nutrients in food rather than increasing them, and makes our food more difficult to digest. Industrial processing depends upon products that have a negative impact on our health, such as refined sugar, white flour, processed and hydrogenated oils, additives, and synthetic vitamins. For example, in the processing of orange juice, the whole orange is put into the machine. Enzymes are added to get as much oil as possible out of the skin. Oranges are very heavily sprayed by chemicals. When they squeeze them, all those pesticides go into the juice that we drink for breakfast ………. brrrr.

To show how commercial agriculture has damaged the food we eat; twenty years ago half pound of fresh spinach contained 50 milligrams of iron, today it contains only 5 milligrams. This same scenario is repeated for every fruit and vegetable produced. By pushing the soil to produce more through the use of chemical pesticides, herbicides, and hormones, the nutrients in the soil have been depleted, and the helpful bacteria and insects destroyed.

Another very toxic substance enhancing food flavors is MSG (monosodium glutamate); it is used in 95% of processed foods. It causes major health problems, including obesity, diseases of the nervous system, cancer, seizures, Alzheimer, and so on. Thing to remember: if it is not in the form God made it, don't eat it. Eliminating processed food, packaged foods, fast food, soda pop, coffee drinks, artificial sweeteners, and all food additives is absolutely crucial.

Processed foods to be avoided include:
- boxed meals (macaroni and cheese, hamburger and tuna 'helpers,' etc.)
- chips and other high-calorie snack foods
- foods made with refined white flour (white breads, pastas, rice)
- frozen dinners
- high-fat canned foods (spaghetti, for example)
- packaged cakes and cookies
- processed meats (sausage, hot dogs, bologna and other packaged lunch meats)
- sodium-laden canned foods
- sugared cereals

If you're planning to wean yourself from convenience foods, start by eliminating processed meats. They're the worst of the worst and are thought to increase your risk of certain types of cancers.

Now about **cooked food**, it puts a strain on our body. To understand why this is true, we need to understand the role enzymes play. Enzymes are in the cells of every living plant and animal. It is enzyme activity that accomplishes all biological work from blinking an eye, to lifting a finger, to having a thought. When we eat, we need enzymes to help digest the food. If the food we eat is raw the enzymes we need are right there in the food itself, ready to go to work for us. If the food is cooked beyond 118 F, these naturally occurring enzymes are killed, and our body must manufacture its own digestive enzymes to do the job.

The father of the food enzyme concept, Dr. Edward Howell, explained that when our body is busy digesting food, it is unable to divert the necessary energy to make the type of enzymes needed to do other tasks. There is a tug-of-war between the demands of our digestive system for a constant supply of digestive enzymes and the needs of our body for the metabolic enzymes vital for cleansing, healing, and building. Without an adequate supply of metabolic enzymes, over time, we suffer.

February 21

Importance of Enzymes

Unfortunately, eating well doesn't always solve the problem. Just because we are eating well doesn't mean that our body is getting the nutrients it needs to thrive. In order to benefit from eating well, our body has to properly digest and absorb the nutrients from the food. The human body produces digestive enzymes that break down the food we eat into nutrients. Nutrients are then absorbed into our body through the small intestine. When we are lacking enzymes, our body doesn't digest properly, and as a result, our body does not absorb the nutrients it needs. A lack of enzymes, along with poor digestion can lead to an overgrowth of parasites, food allergies, unbalanced gut bacteria, constipation, indigestion, gas and bloating and other health issues. Many nutritionists recommend that everyone over the age of thirty five take a daily digestive enzyme supplement.

Enzymes are divided into three main categories: metabolic, digestive, and food enzymes.

Metabolic enzymes catalyze the chemical reaction within the cells of energy production and detoxification. These enzymes are produced by every living microorganism. All the organs, tissues, and cells in our body are dependent on the reaction of metabolic enzymes and their energy factor. Metabolic enzymes actually facilitate our ability to think, feel, see, hear, and move.

Digestive enzymes are responsible for breaking down dietary nutrients and wastes. These enzymes break down the nutrients into their simplest forms in order to be absorbed into the blood stream just as they break down the wastes for expulsion. Most of these enzymes are produced by the body; however, some of these digestive enzymes must be introduced to the body through the raw foods we eat.

Food enzymes are not naturally produced by the body but are just as essential as the ones the body is able to produce. These enzymes need to be introduced to the body through consumption of raw foods. Raw foods naturally contain enzymes, supplying the body with digestive enzymes when ingested. However, raw foods have limited enzymes, not enough to have any support systematically. It only has enough to digest that particular food. Moreover, cooking and processing destroys all of these enzymes, thus, it is recommended that dietary foods are supplemented with enzymes.

Fact: Without enzymes there will be no protection from bacteria, viruses, parasites, yeasts, and others.

February 22

Animal Protein

Dr. T. Colin Campbell, is a researcher who pioneered the investigation of the diet-cancer link in his writings, including "The China Study". This book provides some thought provoking answers to the question 'What really causes cancer?'. One of the biggest contenders: a diet that is higher than 10% animal protein. Here are few facts from this book.

- Population that consumes more animal protein have higher blood cholesterol levels, which in turn are linked to greater rates of heart disease and cancer.
- A high animal protein diet allows more dangerous chemical carcinogens into our cells and facilitates the process by which these carcinogens are transformed by enzymes then bound to our DNA, creating cancer. In experiments, plant protein has been shown to inhibit these processes.
- Women consuming diets high in animal based protein produce greater amounts of reproductive

hormones, which are linked to higher rates of breast cancer.

- Diets high in animal protein have been shown to worsen the formation of kidney stones and draw calcium out of the bones, encouraging osteoporosis.
- Diets that derive most of their protein from a rich variety of unrefined vegetables, legumes, and whole grains have the ability to prevent and sometimes even treat the conditions mentioned above, including heart disease, certain cancers, kidney stones, and osteoporosis.

Dr. Ray Strand, in his book "Healthy for Life" suggests the following sources of protein.

- Best: nuts, avocadoes, olives, beans, soy, and legumes.
- Second best: cold water fish like salmon, mackerel, and sardines.
- Poorest: red meats and dairy products.

Below is a meat comparison table that I found on Dr. Mercola's web site. The meat that he compares is organic and has almost the same amount of protein, but there is a significant difference in amount of calories, fat, and cholesterol. So when we choose to eat meat we should make a smart selection.

Serving (3 oz.)	Calories	Protein (g)	Fat (g)	Chol. (mg)
Ostrich	97	22	2	58
Bison	85	18	2	49
Chicken (skinless)	140	27	3	73
Turkey (skinless)	135	25	3	59
Beef (lean, steak)	240	23	15	77
Pork (lean, loin)	275	24	19	84

February 24

Appointment with Surgeon (Dr. Jane)

I met with Dr. Jane at 2:15pm. We went over the long CAT scan and the tumor and lymph node biopsy reports. There is no indication of lung malignancy, only minor strandy density has developed in the left lung base, presumably atelectasis, nothing to worry about.

The lymph node is clean and cancer is not spreading. However, since it is invasive, the cancerous cells went beyond the tumor's margins and have to be removed. The surgery is scheduled for March 13, Friday.

February 25

Urine Test Results (First)

Today I received the results from the urine test I sent to Philippines on February 11. The number is more than 50, which confirms that I have cancer. When the number changes to 49 or below, I am cured. I will repeat this test in 6 to 8 weeks.

Dear Alexandra,
Your HCG test result on 2-25-09 is:

   Index + 4,(52.2 Int. Units)

This is within the positive range. A positive reading indicates the presence of Human Chorionic Gonadotropin, a hormone found in the urine of pregnant women. Numerous medical reports show this to be present also in the urine of cancer patients. However, the result must be correlated with the medical history together with other pertinent medical information(X-rays, CT Scans, Ultrasounds, MRIs, etc.,). A biopsy procedure confirms the diagnosis of cancer. In reference to the medical history, the result is supportive of the diagnosis of breast cancer. This will serve as the baseline reading.
Wishing you the best of health, I remain
Sincerely yours, EFNavarro,MD

February 26

Probiotic – Importance of Living Bacteria

I forgot to mention that at the beginning of implementing my treatment, I was taking probiotic bacteria VSL#3. I am taking them again. Our immunity begins in the stomach, and most of us have compromised stomach bacteria. One course of antibiotics anytime in our life can permanently change the mix and quantity of these most precious organisms. Probiotic bacterial cultures are intended to assist the body's naturally occurring stomach flora. They are recommended by nutritionists, after a course of antibiotics, or to strengthen the immune system to combat allergies, stress, exposure to toxic substances, and other diseases such as cancer. The August, 2009 issue of the journal Pediatrics contains a study analyzing and confirming the positive effects of probiotics in maintaining immunity and preventing disease. The study also confirmed that probiotic supplementation decreased the length and severity of illness symptoms in those that did get sick. Since about 70% of a person's immune system resides in the glands, mucosa, and mucosa-associated lymphoid system of the gastrointestinal tract, it is vital that the intestinal flora residing in the tract maintain optimal levels and function. Probiotic supplementation is a necessary component to any healthy lifestyle, whether it be through eating cultured and fermented foods like raw milk, kefir, yogurt, miso or kombucha, or through taking probiotic powder, liquid or capsule supplements.

February 27

Organic vs. Not Organic

Here is useful information about organic versus not organic fruits and vegetables. Buying everything organic can be expensive. The Environmental Working Group is a nonprofit organization that protects global and individual health. They provide a Shoppers' Guide to Pesticides in Produce. It is based on the results of nearly 43,000 pesticide tests performed on produce. Of the 43 different fruit and vegetable categories tested, the following foods are divided between '**buy organic**' and '**do not have to be organic**'

Buy Organic	Non-Organic Produce is Okay
Peaches	Onion
Nectarines	Avocado
Berries	Sweet Peas
Apples	Banana
Grapes	Asparagus
Cherries	Cabbage
Carrots	Eggplant
Celery	Sweet Potato
Bell Peppers	Cantaloupe
Spinach	Pineapple
Kale and Collard Greens	Mango
Potatoes	Kiwi Fruit
Lettuce	Watermelon
Pears	Grapefruit
Beets	Broccoli

Complete list is available at www.ewg.org

Fact: Non-organic strawberries are one of the most pesticide-laden fruits available for sale. Organic strawberries contain far more antioxidants, vitamin C and beneficial polyphenolic compounds. Also contain more dry matter per volume, meaning more actual strawberry.

March 1

Mind Control

I enjoy reading Eckhart Tolle. His theories helped me improve my mental condition by learning how to deal with stress. I agree when he says that the true wealth of being can never be found outside of ourselves. The journey toward enlightenment is learning to control our mind. Tolle believes that 80 to 90 percent of our thoughts are not only useless and repetitive, but harmful as well. Our mind is involved continuously in monologues and dialogues, imagining the future based on past events. We worry. We relive the recent or distant past and allow those thoughts and pictures to get in the way of what is real. Tolle believes that we can free our self from the voices. How? Begin by listening, by paying attention to repetitive or compulsive thoughts. As we begin to become aware of our patterns of thinking, we bring in another level of consciousness. Compulsive and repetitive thoughts lose their power over us and we enter a space where we can find an endless source of peace and joy.

Learning to observe the mind allows experiencing the joy of being. Within our mind exist two levels of pain: pain we create now and pain from the past that we continue to identify within the mind and body. The intensity of one's pain is parallel to the degree of resistance to the present moment; therefore, most human pain is unnecessary. To stop creating pain is to stay in the moment, make Now the primary focus in your life. Be careful when the mind has labeled a moment as unpleasant, accept the moment as it is, make it your friend and you will transform your life. As long as we hold on to the pain of past events, negative energy will be created within our mind and body. The more we involve ourselves with the pain, the more pain we create. Tolle believes that Now is the only truly precious thing that matters. Being focused on the past and/or on the future prevents us from Now. This is what I have learned from his 'The Power of Now' book.

The 'Awakening to Your Life's Purpose' book is also very interesting. Here is a powerful story and sentence I found: J. Krishnamurti, the great Indian philosopher spoke and traveled almost continuously all over the world. In the later part of his life he surprised his audience by asking, "Do you want to know my secret?" Everyone became very alert. Many people had been coming to listen to him for twenty or thirty years and still failed to grasp the essence of his teaching. "This is my secret" he said. "I don't mind what happens".

March 2

Living Green: Home Made Cleaning Formulas & Essential Oils

Another change in my life, provoked by the cancer, is reduction of exposure to environmental toxins like pesticides, household chemical cleaners, synthetic air fresheners, and personal products.

Changes that I already made include body soaps, body lotion, deodorant, face lotions, and toothpaste; they all are natural. I also use a natural dishwashing liquid and laundry products.

For many home cleaning chores I started making my own inexpensive cleaning products using formulas listed below. The homemade cleaning formulas cost about one tenth the price of their commercial counterpart.

All purpose cleaner: mix ½ cup vinegar and ¼ cup baking soda into ½ gallon water. Removes water deposit stains, cleans bathroom chrome fixtures, mirrors, etc.
Or
Mix two cups of water, two cups of white vinegar, and few drops of essential oil such as lavender, lemon, or tea tree.

Window cleaner: ¼ - ½ teaspoon natural liquid soap (like dish soap), 2 tablespoons vinegar, 2 cups water, spray bottle

Mold: mix one part hydrogen peroxide with two parts water. Spray and wait an hour. Or use white vinegar or lemon juice full strength.

Carpet stain: use club soda. If stain is tough, use natural soap based carpet cleaner.

Carpet deodorizer: sprinkle baking soda, vacuum in 1/2 hour.

Oven cleaner: mix baking soda with a little of water.

Furniture polish: few drops of lemon or olive oil into ½ cup of warm water. Spray onto a soft cotton cloth.

Wood floors: one quarter cup of white vinegar mixed with 30 ounces of warm water, place it in a spray bottle. This is also good for wood furniture.

Air freshener: keep houseplants, grind lemon in garbage disposal, simmer water and cinnamon or other spices on the stove, bowls of fragrant dried herbs, light a natural candle, burn organic incense.

Clogged sink and bathtub drains: pour a cup of white vinegar plus one cup baking soda into the drain. Let that sit for few moments, flush with teapot full of boiling water. Commercial drain cleaners should never be kept at home, they are the most dangerous.

Essential oils: many people think of essential oils as being useful only for air fresheners, but these oils have antibacterial and antifungal properties that make them great home cleaning products. Not only do they create a pleasing aroma, but they contain no harsh chemicals or artificial additives like commercial disinfectants. Essential oils are multipurpose, friendly to the environment, and safe for your family and pets. However, remember when purchasing oils, look for 'real oils' which you will find in most health food stores, not in the bath or candle shops.

Oils used in home cleaning products:
Lavender, Lime, Pine, Lemon, Grapefruit, Eucalyptus, Orange

Cleaning ways
Using any of the antibacterial oils listed above, place seven drops in a bowl of warm water, and use a clean cloth or sponge to wipe counter tops, tile, and fixtures. Then place two or three drops of Lavender, Thyme, Eucalyptus Lemon, or Tea Tree oil on a separate cloth and wipe doorknobs, faucet handles,

microwave handles, etc. -- these antiviral oils prevent the spread of disease, especially during flu season.

<u>Air Cleansers</u>
Room Spray: Add four or five drops of the oil of your preference to a cup of warm water and pour into a spray bottle. Shake well, and spray in air, or on carpets, furniture, or curtains.
Boiling Water: Placing a few drops of oil in a pot of boiling water removes grease and fat particles from the air in your kitchen, as well as eliminates cooking smells.

Best of all, most of these oils are relatively inexpensive -- around seven to ten dollars per bottle. This may seem like a lot for such a small amount, but remember, you are only using a few drops at a time.

How to Remove Pesticides from Produce
We all know about them - pesticides and waxes that cover our produce. Although there are many fruit and vegetable washes available in supermarkets, it's simple to make your own homemade blend that will work just as well and at a fraction of the cost.

<u>Consider these facts:</u>
- Bacteria and fungus occur naturally on most crops. Even if there is no visible soil clinging to your non-organic or organic produce, bacteria can be present.
- Imagine how many hands touch the food before it gets to your mouth, plus bacteria from soil and dirt can accumulate during the shipping process: these can cause a buildup on the surface of any produce.
- Agriculture pesticides are not removable with water alone.

Produce Wash 1
- 20 drops grapefruit seed extract, available at health food stores
- 1 Tablespoon baking soda
- 1 cup white vinegar
- 1 cup water
- New spray bottle

Produce Wash 2
- 1 Tablespoon lemon juice

- 1 Tablespoon white vinegar
- 1 cup water
- New spray bottle

Spray produce. Let sit 5-10 minutes and rinse thoroughly to wash away residue.

NOTE: The baking soda and vinegar will foam when mixed together. Make sure you use a deep pitcher and pour slowly.

March 3

Alkaline and Acidic Foods Table

Otto Warburg discovered the mechanism of cancer cells during the 1930s. He received a Nobel Prize for his discovery. When cells are no longer metabolizing with oxygen they go from respiration to fermentation, this is why sugar should be forbidden.

One of the most important actions in the battle with cancer is eliminating acidic foods. In addition to removing oxygen from our cells, they create mucus in the body, and mucus acts like glue, clogging our elimination organs. Also acidity lowers the pH of the body, creating an environment for cancer cells to thrive in. Excess acidity is a condition that weakens all body systems. Excess acidity forces the body to borrow minerals – including calcium, sodium, potassium and magnesium – from vital organs and bones to buffer (neutralize) the acid and safely remove it from the body.

Anything that is acidic or toxic will force our body to work overtime, parking the acidic waste into cells, producing more cholesterol, and leaching our needed minerals to neutralize the acids.

Almost all foods that we eat, after being digested, absorbed, and metabolized, release either an acid or an alkaline base into the blood. Grains, fish, meat, poultry, shellfish, cheese, milk, and salt all produce acid, so the introduction and dramatic rise in our consumption of these foods meant that the typical Western diet became more acid-producing. Consumption of fresh fruit and vegetables decreased, which further made the Western diet acid-producing.

Regardless of how much we work out and try to eat right, if we can't balance the acids in our body, we'll never feel as good as we would like to be. When acidic wastes accumulate, they can cause organs to malfunction and break down. This creates a fertile breeding ground for various forms of chronic illness that are now experienced by more than half the population.

If we often feel tired, it's a safe bet that we are overly acidic. The simple fact is, most people are.

Our blood is slightly alkaline, with a normal pH level of between 7.35 and 7.45. The theory behind the alkaline diet is that our diet should reflect this pH level (as it did in the past) and be slightly alkaline. Proponents of alkaline diets believe that a diet high in acid-producing foods disrupts this balance and promotes the loss of essential minerals. This imbalance is thought to make people prone to illness.

Dr. Theodore Baroody, author of "Alkalize or Die" says:

"The countless names of illnesses do not really matter. What does matter is that they all come from the same basic root cause ...... too much acid tissue waste in the body!"

According to Sang Whang, author of "Reverse Aging", Even if we eat the best of organic fruit and vegetables, 97% of our food still consists of carbon, nitrogen, hydrogen and oxygen, which will still be reduced to acid waste. He says that it is not what we put into our bodies ... it's what stays in our bodies as waste that creates our over acidic condition and causes us to age prematurely and get ill.

To make it easy, here are a few highly alkaline foods that would go a long way towards improving the diet. Consider adding paprika, parsley and horseradish, squeeze lemon or lime juice on fish, salads, or in your beverage. Add onions to everything. Munch on pumpkin seeds, or add them to the salad. Use sea salt (Celtic, French or Himalayan preferred) avoid

34

regular table salt. Substitute sweet potatoes for red potatoes. Use Apple cider vinegar rather than Balsamic vinegar. Choose miso soup with seaweed. Add crushed ginger to your morning eggs and other foods. If you like radishes, eat them like candy. If you want something sweet, eat unsweetened pineapple, mango, cantaloupe, tangerines, mandarin oranges, kiwi and assorted berries. Let watermelon or vegetable juice be your summer thirst quencher. Control a hunger with celery smeared with nut butter. Smear half of an avocado on toast, rather than margarine. Add asparagus, winter squash and chestnuts to round out the list of extreme alkaline foods.

The following table is helpful in understanding which foods to eat and which once to avoid.

Healthy Alkaline Foods - Eat lots of them!	Foods you should only consume moderately	Unhealthy Acidic Foods - Try to avoid them!
Vegetables	*Fruits*	*Meat, Poultry, And Fish*
Alfalfa Grass +29.3	*In Season, With Moderation*	Beef -34.5
Asparagus +1.3	Apricot -9.5	Chicken -18.0
Barley Grass +28.1	Bananna, Ripe -10.1	Liver -3.0
Brussels Sprouts +0.5	Bananna, Unripe +4.8	Ocean Fish -20.0
Cabbage Lettuce +14.1	Black Currant -6.1	Organ Meats -3.0
Cauliflower +3.1	Blueberry -5.3	Oysters -5.0
Cayenne Pepper +18.8	Cantaloupe -2.5	Pork -38.0
Celery +13.3	Cherry, Sour +3.5	Veal -35.0
Chives +8.3	Cherry, Sweet -3.6	
Cucumber, Fresh +31.5	Coconut, Fresh +0.5	*Milk And Milk Products*
Dandelion +22.7	Cranberry -7.0	Buttermilk +1.3
Garlic +13.2	Currant -8.2	Cream -3.9
Green Cabbage +4.0	Date -4.7	Hard Cheese -18.1
Leeks (Bulbs) +7.2	Fig Juice Powder -2.4	Homogenized Milk -1.0
Lettuce +2.2	Gooseberry, Ripe -7.7	Quark -17.3
Onion +3.0	Grape, Ripe -7.6	
Peas, Fresh +5.1	Grapefruit -1.7	*Bread, Biscuits*
Red Cabbage +6.3	Italian Plum -4.9	Rye Bread -2.5
Rhubarb Stalks +6.3	Mandarin Orange -11.5	White Biscuit -6.5
Savoy Cabbage +4.5	Mango -8.7	White Bread -10.0
Soy Sprouts +29.5	Orange -9.2	Whole-Grain Bread -4.5
Spinach +13.1	Papaya -9.4	Whole-Meal Bread -6.5
Watercress +7.7	Peach -9.7	
Wheat Grass +33.8	Pear -9.9	*Nuts*
White Cabbage +3.3	Pineapple -12.6	Cashews -9.3
Zucchini +5.7	Rasberry -5.1	Peanuts -12.8
	Red Currant -2.4	Pistachios -16.6

Root Vegetables
Beet +11.3
Carrot +9.5
Horseradish +6.8
Potatoes +2.0
Red Radish +16.7
Black Radish +39.4
Turnip +8.0
White Radish +3.1

Fruits
Avocado (Protein) +15.6
Fresh Lemon +9.9
Limes +8.2
Tomato +13.6

Grains And Legumes
Buckwheat +0.5
Lentils +0.6
Lima Beans +12.0
Soy Flour +2.5
Soybeans, Fresh +12.0
Spelt +0.5
Tofu +3.2
White Beans +12.1

Nuts
Almonds +3.6
Brazil Nuts +0.5

Seeds
Cumin Seeds +1.1
Fennel Seeds +1.3
Flax Seeds +1.3
Pumpkin Seeds +5.6
Sesame Seeds +0.5
Sunflower Seeds +5.4

Fats (Fresh, Cold-Pressed Oils)
Borage Oil +3.2
Evening Primrose Oil +4.1
Flax Seed Oil +3.5
Olive Oil +1.0

Rose Hips -15.5
Strawberry -5.4
Tangerine -8.5
Watermelon -1.0
Yellow Plum -4.9

Grains
Brown Rice -12.5
Wheat -10.1

Nuts
Hazelnuts -2.0
Macadamia Nuts -3.2
Walnuts -8.0

Fish
Fresh Water Fish -11.8

Fats
Coconut Milk -1.5
Sunflower Oil -6.7

Fats
Butter -3.9
Corn Oil -6.5
Margarine -7.5

Sweets
Artificial Sweetners -26.5
Barley Malt Syrup -9.3
Beet Sugar -15.1
Chocolate -24.6
Molasses -14.6
White Sugar -17.6

Condiments
Ketchup -12.4
Mayonaise -12.5
Mustard -19.2
Soy Sauce -36.2
Vinegar -39.4

Beverages
Beer -26.8
Coffee -25.1
Fruit Juice, Natural -8.7
Liquor -38.7
Tea (Black) -27.1
Wine -16.4

Miscellaneous
Canned Foods
Microwaved Foods
Processed Foods

Table: pH scale of alkaline and acid forming foods
(Source: "Back To The House Of Health" by Shelley Redford Young)

Inexpensive tricks for Higher Alkalinity
- Half teaspoon of baking soda (not baking powder) with warm water before bed time. Try this in two weeks stretches with a week off.
- Warm water with freshly squeezed lemon upon waking up.

March 4

Where to Look for Alkaline Water
How Safe is Fluoride

For the first time, since I started to take 94 tables a day, something felt wrong. For two days I felt pain in my belly, I felt locked up, and very uncomfortable. I wasn't sure what was happening to me. I looked back trying to identify recent changes made to my cancer program. Bingo! I have upgraded the type of the fiber that I am taking from an average to Fiberzon made by Amazon Herb Co. Fiberzon is much more potent, made out of pure blends of organic Rainforest herbs. I made a phone call and was reminded that every time I take Fiberzon I need to drink at least a full glass of water. Once I heard this I drank 4 glasses and my pain was gone! I felt so relieved!

Lesson #1; while taking several servings of supplements a day make sure that each serving is supported by at least 1 full glass of water, which means I will be drinking at least 8 glasses a day! If this is the case I better make sure I drink the best water!

I have a Reverse Osmosis Drinking Water System; this water is not alkaline, ionized, and oxygenated enough. However, unlike most carbon filter systems, reverse osmosis will actually remove the fluoride that most U.S. municipalities add to their water. Reverse osmosis will remove virtually all contaminants from the water, including fluoride, especially when combined with a pre- and post-carbon filtration system.

For a while now I am thinking about purchasing an ionizer and alkaline rejuvenating water machine. Since this is between a

37

$1,000 and $1,500 investment I want to make sure that I pick the right one for my needs. I studied four most popular ionizers available today; Tyent, Jupiter, Life Ionizer, and Enagic. The Life Ionizer seems to be the most popular, given its affordability and the quality of water. However, later I read that the famous doctor that helped make electrolysis-ionizers so popular in the early 1980's (Dr. Hidemitsu Hayashi) continued his research and later determined that the health benefits of ionized water observed in clinical studies are a result of the hydrogen content in the freshly created water. More troubling to him was that the 'home' versions of these ionizers typically create water so slowly that all the hydrogen has evaporated out before enough water has been created to drink! This makes it impossible for most to consume enough hydrogen-rich water throughout the day, even if one owns an electrolysis-ionizer.

Dr. Hidemitsu Hayashi recently invented a new way to create alkaline, ionized, hydrogen-rich water without any of the above problems using magnesium and far-infrared ceramics. The 'Hydrogen-Rich Water Stick' is simply kept in water bottle and continually produces hydrogen-rich water to be consumed anywhere for six months. Because I have cancer, I need a potent amount of alkaline, ionized, and anti-oxidant water, so I have purchased two sticks.

Fact: A good way to start the day is drinking 'good' water with freshly squeezed lemon juice; it helps detoxify the liver and alkalize the body

How safe is fluoride?
Fluoride is one of the most toxic substances known to man. Most European countries have banned its use. Yet it is in most brands of toothpaste for preventative dental care. Other products, such as bottled water, infant formulas, and even vitamin supplements, now contain fluoride. Ironically, the fluoride has never been proven to significantly aid in protecting teeth from the development of cavities. Fluoride poisoning severely damages the body and can be fatal. This lethal chemical creates a toxic state that can cause a variety of harmful effects. All of the beverages sold in stores use tap water. The customers who drink those beverages ingest a fair amount of added fluoride. When the availability of such

beverages is combined with the amount of fluoridated tap water, one can appreciate the high level of fluoride in the present-day diet.

Fluoride is a soluble salt, not a heavy metal. There are two basic types of fluoride. Calcium fluoride appears naturally in underground water sources and even seawater. Enough of it can cause skeletal or dental fluorosis, which weakens bone and dental matter. But it is not nearly as toxic, nor does it negatively affect so many other health issues as sodium fluoride, which is added to many water supplies.

Sodium Fluoride is a synthetic waste product of the nuclear, aluminum, and phosphate fertilizer industries. This fluoride has an amazing capacity to combine and increase the potency of other toxic materials. It damages the liver and kidneys, weakens the immune system, possibly leading to cancer.

With that being said, the great news is—the human body can detoxify and repair itself at a rapid rate. So it's not too late to cleanse our body and begin avoiding this toxic chemical!

Liver Cleanses are considered effective for eliminating fluorides and other toxins. Also taking a lot of vitamin C and adding calcium and magnesium supplements with plenty of pure water, good sleep and rest, and the detox should be relatively smooth.

March 7

Why Multivitamins and Minerals are Important
Difference Between Synthetic and Natural Vitamins
How to Read Labels

With the soil being so depleted, the air so polluted, less oxygen in the air and less sunlight hitting the earth we need to take more amounts of nutrients today than those who lived even a hundred years ago. The fact that our food is also about ten times less nutritious than it was a hundred years makes taking a good whole food multivitamin that much more important. Multivitamins and supplements ensure that we are getting a healthy dose of specific vitamins.

What is the difference between synthetic and natural vitamins?

Many vitamin and mineral supplements are manufactured synthetically with chemicals and do not come straight from their natural sources and are not meant for human consumption. Evolution has dictated that we eat the food we can gather from the earth, not the food we create in a lab! There are many negative health and environmental impacts from synthetic ingredients in vitamins and supplements. Put simply, the human body has evolved for millions of years to digest foods found in nature. Most synthetically produced vitamins and supplements are chemical compounds that cannot be found in nature; therefore the human body does not recognize these ingredients which can result in unanticipated reactions. The body knows the difference between real and fake and it always prefers real.

How can we check what companies to trust?

Over the next few months, the Organic Consumers Association will be building a list of vitamin/supplement producers that ranks them based on criteria that assesses how close that product is to being 100% organic and naturally occurring. If you have a specific brand of vitamin/supplement that your are curious about, you can submit that company to http://www.organicconsumers.org/nutricon/nutripetition.cfm, and they will investigate its ingredients.

Another way to check if you are buying good product is by utilizing the 'Comparative Guide to Nutritional Supplements'. This guide compares 500 products made by 213 companies. You can check if the company that you are using is in the 150 bottom. If it is I suggest switching. The guide is available in www.comparativeguide.com.

Fact: Did you know that 95% of all vitamin supplements sold today fall in to the synthetic category? Did you know that most vitamins on the market claiming to be natural are only 10% natural! If you decide to buy natural, it is important you learn to read labels to assure receiving your money's worth.

Here is a table that helps determine whether your vitamins are natural or synthetic:

Item:	If source Given Is:	It Is:
Vitamin A	Fish Oils	Natural Co-Natural
	Lemon Grass	Natural
	Acetate	Synthetic
	Palmitate	Synthetic
	If source not given	Synthetic
Vitamin B-Complex	Brewers Yeast	Natural
	If source not given	Synthetic
Vitamin B1 (Thiamine)	Yeast	Natural
	Thiamine Mononitrate	Synthetic
	Thiamine Hydrochloride	Synthetic
Vitamin B2 (Riboflavin)	Yeast	Natural
	Riboflavin	Synthetic
Pantothenic Acid	Yeast, Rice Bran or Liver	Natural
	Calcium D-Pantothenate	Synthetic
Vitamin B6 (Pyridoxine)	Yeast	Natural
	Pyridoxine Hydrochloride	Synthetic
Vitamin B12	Liver	Natural Co-Natural
	Micro-organism fermentation	Co-Natural
	Cobalamin Concentrate	Co-Natural
PABA	Yeast - Para-aminobenzoic Acid	Natural
	Aminobenzoic Acid	Synthetic
Folic Acid	Yeast or Liver	Natural
	Pteroylglutamic Acid	Synthetic
Inositol	Soy Beans	Natural Co-Natural
	Reduced from Corn	Co-Natural
Choline	Soy Beans	Natural
	Choline Chloride	Synthetic
	Choline Bitartrate	Synthetic
Biotin	Liver	Natural
	d-Biotin	Synthetic
Niacin	Yeast	Natural Co-Natural
	Niacinamide	Co-Natural
	Niacin	Synthetic

Vitamin C (Ascorbic Acid)	Citrus, Rose Hips, Acerola Berries	Natural
	Ascorbic Acid	Synthetic
	If source not given	Synthetic
Vitamin D	Fish Oils	Natural
	Irradiated Ergosteral (Yeast)	Synthetic
	Calciferol	Synthetic
Vitamin E	Veg Oil, Wheat Germ Oil, or Mixed Tocopherols	Natural
		Natural
	d-alpha tocopherol	Natural
	dl-alpha tocopherol (any "dl-" forms)	Synthetic
Vitamin F	Essential Fatty Acids	Natural
Vitamin K	Alfalfa	Natural
	Menadione	Synthetic

Vitamin is an organic compound that is necessary for normal growth and maintenance of life. Vitamins fall into two categories: fat soluble and water soluble. The fat-soluble vitamins — A, D, E, and K — dissolve in fat and can be stored in our body. The water-soluble vitamins — C and the B-complex vitamins (such as vitamins B6 or B12) — need to dissolve in water before our body can absorb them. Because of this, our body can't store these vitamins. Any vitamin C or B that our body doesn't use as it passes through our system is lost (mostly when we pee). So we need a fresh supply of these vitamins every day.

Some vitamins:
A (Natural beta-carotene) – healthy vision, skin and immune system, guards infections
C – promotes tissue growth and repair, healthy gums, guards heart
E – supports muscular system, overall joint health, antioxidant, protects DNA
D's – healthy bone density, healthy teeth, protects DNA, fights cancer
K – proper bone and blood function
B12 – energy production, for more see May 16

While vitamins are organic substances (made by plants or animals), **minerals** are inorganic elements that come from the soil and water and are absorbed by plants or eaten by animals. A mineral is a naturally occurring solid formed through geological processes that has a characteristic chemical composition. They are essential for human metabolism. They are involved in responses of the nervous system and muscles, the absorption and emission of the body's fluids, and maintain a delicate water balance within the body.

Some minerals:
Calcium – provides high level of support for our skeletal system, most abundant in our body
Chromium – supports normal blood sugar levels
Copper – to process iron
Iron – transport of oxygen thru blood
Iodine – normal cell metabolism, involved in production of thyroid hormones, necessary for proper growth
Magnesium – promotes bone density, maintains muscular and nervous system, supports healthy heart, supports lungs and overall pulmonary system
Potassium – promotes bone density, regulates circulatory system and promotes hearth health
Selenium – supports immune system, antioxidant, fights breast cancer
Zinc – process protein into energy, maintain vision, boost immunity, fights breast cancer
Boron – healthy bone density

Precautions to consider when mixing certain nutrients:
- In higher doses, vitamin C can destroy vitamin B-12; they should be taken at a different time of day.
- The flavonoids in vegetables normally block iron absorption, but vitamin C dramatically increases the absorption of iron, even in the presence of vegetables. If you are concerned with reducing iron, take vitamin C between meals; if you need more iron take it with meals.
- The iron in meats is highly absorbable but can be blocked by vegetables, so meat should be eaten with vegetables to reduce iron, which increases risk of cancer, and worsen great number of other illnesses, such as diabetes and arthritis.

March 9

Buckwheat (Kasha)
Quinoa

A few times a week my menu includes **buckwheat** or quinoa, and I love it. Buckwheat's name is deceiving; it is not wheat, but seed. Buckwheat has numerous health benefits. It does not contain gluten; studies have indicated that consuming buckwheat fights high blood pressure and high cholesterol; Buckwheat does not lead to peaks in blood sugar levels, three servings per day lowers diabetes 26%. Buckwheat supports the body's healing and inhibits cancer, it increases immune boosting friendly bacteria. It contains a full spectrum of essential amino acids, making it one of the few vegetarian sources of complete protein that equals the protein of fish or meat in quality.

Remember, toasted buckwheat which has a golden brown color, tastes the best. The raw buckwheat is white or light green. If you buy raw buckwheat you should toast it yourself; toss it lightly in a dry skillet over medium heat until it colors. Buckwheat is available in the specialty grocers carrying European foods, you can find it in whole foods stores as well. In Austin, go to Sasha's, Phoenicia or Sun Harvest.

Buckwheat is easy to prepare: one portion of brown buckwheat with two portions of drinking water, add tablespoon of olive oil and sea salt for taste. Bring it to boil, reduce heat to minimum, cook it for another 10 minutes or until all seeds are separate. Keep it covered all the time.

Buckwheat is very versatile; you can include it in salads, with sweet or savory dishes. You can eat it by itself, or combine it with anything you wish. Buckwheat is popular in Northern Europe, traditionally served as an accompaniment to meats. For example, a quick snack includes cooked buckwheat, avocado, a dash of olive oil, and sea salt. Here is another good way to prepare it:

1. Soak dried mushrooms, such as shitake, in two cups of drinking water until soft.

2. Drain, saving the soaking water, and slice discarding any tough portions.
3. Add one cup of brown buckwheat to soaking liquid and bring it to boil.
4. Lower heat and add carrot, onion, and mushrooms.
5. Cover and simmer until water is absorbed. Add sea salt to taste.

Quinoa (pronounced keen-wah), same as buckwheat, is not a grain, it is a seed. When cooked, quinoa is light, fluffy, slightly crunchy and subtly flavored. It actually cooks and tastes like a grain, making it an excellent replacement for grains that are difficult to digest or feed candida (a systemic fungal infection).

Some of the nutrients in quinoa include:
- Complete protein. Quinoa contains all 9 essential amino acids that are required by the body as building blocks for muscles.
- Magnesium helps relax your muscles and blood vessels and effects blood pressure. Quinoa contains high levels of this vital nutrient.
- Fiber. Quinoa is a wonderful way to ensure that you consume valuable fiber that eases elimination and tones your colon.
- Manganese and copper. Quinoa is a good source of these minerals that act as antioxidants in your body to get rid of dangerous cancer and disease-causing substances.

Quinoa, in its whole grain form, may be effective in preventing and treating these conditions:
- Artherosclerosis
- Breast cancer
- Diabetes
- Insulin resistance

Quinoa is close to one of the most complete foods in nature because it contains amino acids, enzymes, vitamins and minerals, fiber, antioxidants, and phytonutrients. Quinoa does not feed fungal and bacterial infections in your body (and doctors estimate that 8 in 10 Americans have fungal infections, like candida!).

Quinoa has other qualities that make it an ideal "grain":
- Quinoa acts as a probiotic that feeds the microflora (good bacteria) in your intestines.
- Quinoa is easily digested for optimal absorption of nutrients.
- Quinoa is gluten-free and safe for those with gluten intolerance, people on a celiac diet, and for autistic children who follow the Body Ecology program for autism.

Here are some ideas for your quinoa meal:
- Sautee garlic, onions, and spinach with oil to top your quinoa.
- Make a summery salad by chopping raw carrots, zucchini, cultured vegetables, and onions over quinoa.
- Use quinoa with vegetable broth and your choice of vegetables for a nutritious soup.
- Top quinoa with salsa, use recipe from May 3.

Buckwheat and quinoa are a very inexpensive addition to my menu and I love it!

Ways to save money on food include:

1. Eat at home.
   Recent study reported that meals consumed at home cost about a third of those purchased away from home. This choice alone saves $66 of every $100 in the food budget and you control what you eat.
2. Take it with you.
   Pack your lunch. Have healthy snacks available; a bag of almonds or pumpkin seeds. Do not leave the house without water in a reusable container.
3. Buy wisely.
   Processed foods, including frozen and baked goods, claim over 40% of total supermarket sales while fruits and vegetables represent 9%. Buy in bulk.
4. Eat seasonally.
   Purchase locally grown produce items in season. Grow your own. Connect with area producers.

46

March 11

Tooth Extraction
Mercury and Calcium Bentonite Clay

This morning Dr. David extracted the root canal tooth that was infected. I have been trying to schedule this important procedure for few weeks and am very happy that this is behind me. I was convinced that this tooth had major impact on my process of healing and I couldn't wait to get rid of it. Now I should heal more quickly and with more profound results. Teeth are connected to different body organs, it is important to keep our month in impeccable condition, so the rest of the body is not affected.

The second action on my list is to remove the couple of silver fillings still left in my mouth; these fillings are 50% mercury. Mercury is a powerful poison, the most toxic, non radioactive element on the earth. The International Academy of Medicine and Toxicology believes we should have mercury fillings removed. Mercury vapor is continuously emitted from dental fillings and accumulates in the body over time. Studies repeatedly demonstrate that even low levels of mercury cause measurable health effects. To prevent mercury exposure it is recommended to find a biological dentist properly trained in mercury filling removal. In Austin I found only four dentists with such qualifications: Dr. Griffin Cole, Dr. Joan Sefcik, Dr. Merrily Sandford, and Dr. Sasi K. Mannem.

While having the fillings removed there is a new protocol being recognized by the alternative naturopathic health practitioners that uses **Calcium Bentonite Clay for detoxing mercury** from the body. The Clay is able to extract heavy metals, radioactive elements and many other toxins such as pesticides from the body. To understand more about the remarkable abilities of healing clay go to www.AboutClay.com. They recommend 2 clay baths a week for 5 weeks using 2 cups of Therapeutic Living Clay per bath. Since Mercury tends to linger it would not hurt to repeat clay baths twice a year. The beauty of clay is that it draws impurities to itself and pulls them into itself so that danger of re-absorption by the body is not likely to occur. Some products loosen the metals so to speak but are not as good at capturing them like clay.

Additional principles related dental health:

- Root canals: Be cautious of root canals as they can have many adverse consequences for your health. They collect toxins.
- Crowns: Avoid ceramic and porcelain crowns as they have metal in them. Request composites.
- Sealants: Avoid dental sealants for children, as they contain potent cancer-causing xenoestrogens. Many also contain high levels of fluoride.
- Avoid fluoride. It should not be used in your toothpaste, water, as a supplement, or in your dental office. Fluoride is a metabolic poison and will actually damage your teeth.

One of the simple ways to detox the body is cilantro. Cilantro not only tastes great, it also binds to heavy metals and helps remove them from the body. This is potentially a life-saving product; add it to your meals.

Finally, mercury does not come only from the dental fillings; we also get it from the flu and other vaccines and fish. The typical rule of thumb when considering fish consumption: the larger the fish, the more mercury in it. It was proven that the Alaskan Wild Red Salmon is our best choice.

Fact: Only enzymes, nutrition, and lifestyle provide health care. Drugs only provide disease and symptoms management, not cure.

Fact: Majority of all cancer comes from environmental pollution; chemically tainted foods we eat, the air we breathe, and the water we drink.

Fact: When people don't get enough minerals from their food, the body is forced to steal it from the bones, leading to osteoporosis.

| Lowest Mercury | Lower Mercury | High Mercury | Highest Mercury |
6-oz per week	6-oz per month	6-os per month	AVOID EATING
Anchovies	Carp	Bass saltwater	Grouper
Bitterfish	Mahi Mahi	Croaker	Marlin
Calamari (squid)	Crab	Halibut	Orange roughy
Caviar	Snapper	Tuna	Tilefish
Pollok	Crab	Sea treout	Swordfish
Catfish	Herring	Bluefish	Shark
Whitefish	Monkfish	Lobster	Mackrel king
Perch (ocean)	Perach		
Scallops	Skate		
Flounder	Cod		
Haddock	Tuna		
Hake			
Shad			
Sole			
Crafish			
Salmon			
Shrimp			
Clams			
Tilapia			
Oysters			
Sardines			
Trout			

Chart obtained from the Natural Resource Defense Council (NRDC)

March 13

Second Breast Surgery

Today is Friday the 13th, my lucky day. This morning, at 5:30 am, I went to hospital for the second breast surgery. This time I considered myself experienced. It was much easier to deal with the pre-surgery procedures. First I had to pay for my portion of the surgery. Next they took me to my private room, very clean and comfortable. I removed all my clothes, slipped into the hospital gown, and laid down on a mobile bed under a few layers of blankets. The first nurse showed up to check my vital signs, then another nurse came to attach an IV in my vein. After that the Anesthesiologist came to talk about the upcoming procedure, when he left his nurse came to check the IV and to tell me that the injection will start soon. Then my doctor came, she said that she is ready for the surgery and asked if I had any questions. Then they took me to the surgery room. I was out before we reached the destination. When I woke up I was back in my hospital room. Dr. Jane had already talked to my Mom; the surgery went well, the biopsy results will be available this Tuesday. As before, my chest was tidily wrapped with bandages that I was told to keep on for 24 hours, no showers allowed. On my way home I felt no pain, I was glad the surgery was over.

Later I had to take pain medication, it wasn't because of the breast pain, it was because of my tooth removal. The tooth surgery happened to be more traumatic than the breast surgery. Interesting.........

I checked the cut on my breast; it is just a little larger than the one from before, the shape and size of my breast has changed a little, now it has a cavity in it.

March 16

Food Combining
Ice-cold foods or beverages

In my case, the uncomfortable side affect of being on the raw vegetable diet is gas and bloating. Feeling this way made me anxious to find out what I can do to stop it. Change in diet is NOT an option. Besides, I like my diet, even now, over a month of being very strict about it.

This is how I came across the food combining theory. This theory is based on the fact that each type of food required different lengths of time, different enzymes and different degree of acidity or alkalinity for proper digestion. In addition, incomplete digestion forces the body to spend more energy creating more digestive enzymes, robbing it of the energy it needs to create tissue building, metabolic enzymes.

Once I got familiar with the food combining theory I realized that my gas and bloating is not caused by the wrong food combinations. I eat mostly raw vegetables, gluten free bread and buckwheat, and watch the acidic foods. My food combination is very simple, mostly vegetables with vegetables. So my issue is still unresolved. I bet the main reason is that I eat raw vegetables as 80% of my daily intake, which until now my body was not use to. Every change needs an adjustment time. I need to continue my research to find more educated answers.

Each type of food, proteins, carbohydrates, and fats require a different internal environment in our system for proper digestion. Carbs are mainly digested in our small intestine, and require an alkaline environment. Proteins require a more acidic environment and are mainly broken down in the stomach.

When we eat carbs and proteins together, these contradicting requirements can delay the digestion of both. This in turn could let the carbs ferment and the proteins ROT, right in our stomach!

I found good information in the book ' Health begins in the colon' by Dr. Group. Dr. Group follows these guidelines in his life and with his patients:

- Do not eat starches and proteins in the same meal
- Do not combine starches with acidic foods such as fruit juices and vinegar
- Do not combine proteins with acidic foods such as fruit
- Do not eat meat with milk or cheese

When these combinations of foods are eaten, the digestive process is disturbed and incomplete digestion takes place. This leaves toxic waste behind in the intestines.

Rules for healthy diet include:

- Combine proteins with non-starchy vegetables
- Eat a diet consisting of 80% alkaline foods, such as vegetables and fruits (even fruits that may seem acidic, like lemon, will turn alkaline in the digestive tract)
- Eat 5 balanced meals each day

Following are meal suggestions for a typical day.

Breakfast: Eat between 4am and 9 am; eat fruit or drink fruit juice, choose a variety of fruits during a week. Don't mix sweet fruits (bananas, melons, peaches) with acid fruits (citrus, strawberries, kiwis, sour apples). It is also good to have flaxseed oil with organic cottage cheese; see April 1st.

Mid-morning snack: Eat halfway between breakfast and lunch; good choices include raw nuts or seeds, goji berries, or avocado with lime and pepper.

Lunch: Eat between 11:30am and 1:30pm; choose a starch and vegetables plus salad; good starches include grains, potatoes, Ezekiel bread, and squashes; good vegetables will be alkaline such as dark green and orange ones.

Mid-afternoon snack: Eat half way between lunch and dinner; choose one of the options listed for the mid-morning snack but a different option from the one eaten earlier.

Dinner: Eat between 6pm and 8pm; eat a large vegetable salad sprinkled with some high quality oil followed by a protein source such as fish, cheese, eggs, if necessary organic meat. Sea salt or Braggs Amino Acids may provide some flavor.

Here is the food combining chart for reference.

Food Combining Simplified

One food at a meal is the most ideal for the easiest and best digestion.
A combination of several foods at a meal should be according to the chart below.

Proteins ⇐ [Poor Combination] ⇒ Hi-Starches

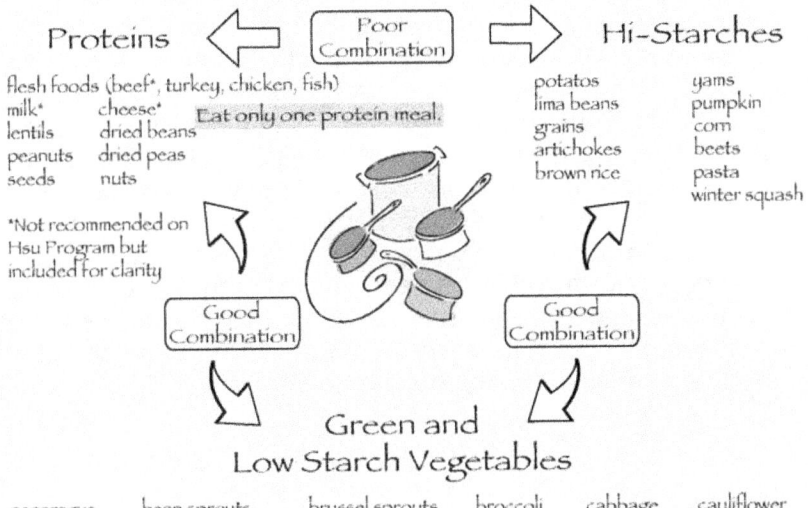

Proteins		Hi-Starches	
flesh foods (beef*, turkey, chicken, fish)		potatos	yams
milk*	cheese*	lima beans	pumpkin
lentils	dried beans	grains	corn
peanuts	dried peas	artichokes	beets
seeds	nuts	brown rice	pasta
			winter squash

Eat only one protein meal.

*Not recommended on Hsu Program but included for clarity

[Good Combination]   [Good Combination]

Green and Low Starch Vegetables

asparagus	bean sprouts	brussel sprouts	broccoli	cabbage	cauliflower
celery	cucumbers	eggplant	endive	escarole	leaf lettuce
greens	leeks	kohlrabi	mushrooms	okra	olives
peppers	radishes	rhubarb	sauerkraut	spinach	string beans
summer squash		swiss chard	watercress	sea vegetables	

Tomatos may be combined with low-starch vegetables and either nuts or avocados.

Avocados are best combined with low-starch vegetables.
(They make a "fair" combination with starches.)

Eat only fresh fruits for breakfast

Eat only one kind of fruit at a time, as much as you want.
Wait one hour, then eat another kind, if you so desire.
Stop one hour before lunch.
Melons are best eaten alone.

Advice to remember: avoid ice-cold foods or beverages as they can damage the nerve endings of the stomach. A hand, held in icy water, becomes numb. Similarly, cold drinks or food items cause the stomach cells to bond and prevent them from producing the required amounts of digestive juices. They also make the stomach insensitive to potentially harmful foods or beverages, and effectively disrupt its communication and potential warning signals to the brain. In addition, digestive enzymes require a very specific temperature to operate optimally. By cooling down the enzymes' environment, their digestive and anti-cancer properties begin to diminish, predisposing a person to excessive weight gain and even cancer. Also, the sudden cold influence, as caused, for example, by ice cream or iced beverages, forces the body to increase its internal heat generation in order to compensate for the harmful drop in temperature. This response wastes the body's energy reserves and makes it feel even hotter and thirstier than before, particularly during the summer period. Foods and beverages that are of room temperature or warm are the most suitable and natural ones for the human body.

March 19

Second Surgery Biopsy Results

Second breast surgery biopsy results are still positive, the margins are not clear again, my cancer continues to be 'invasive ductal adenocarcinoma' type. I met with Dr. Jane today; she said that I have two options: have another breast lumpectomy re-excision or remove the entire breast and have a reconstruction at the same time. I have decided to have another excision.

I have learned that women with breast cancer who undergo lumpectomy could avoid a return trip to the operating room, thanks to laboratory test done during the surgery that quickly confirms whether surgeons have removed all cancerous cells or not. This method is known as frozen section analysis. Unfortunately this does not work with my type of cancer, I will have to relay on Dr. Jane's skills and luck.

The next surgery is scheduled for April 14, which gives me almost a month for continuing my natural way of healing. Once my cells get healthy, the cancer will be kicked out of my system.

Dr. Jane suggested that I meet with an Oncologist. I told her that I made a decision not to do the chemo therapy; she understood, however she asked that I make an appointment anyway to learn about it and perhaps to go thru more tests for the purpose of identifying the cancer with more detail. I was referred to Dr. Beth, apparently one of the best Oncologists in town, I am checking her references.

I keep repeating the reasons why I want to avoid chemotherapy: when the body has too much toxic burden from chemo and radiation the immune system is either compromised or destroyed, we are open to various infections and complications. Chemo and radiation cause cancer cells to mutate and become resistant and difficult to destroy. Unfortunately surgery can also cause cancer cells to spread; however, I have chosen surgery because I had to make a decision right away. The information I have today was not available to me that day and doctors were not telling me about any other way of healing besides surgery, radiation, and chemotherapy.

March 26

Appointment with Oncologist

This morning I met with Dr. Beth, the oncologist recommended by Dr. Jane. She explained the program I should undertake, she also answered several of my questions. The bottom line is that she has no doubt that I need to take some kind of chemotherapy, the kind will be based on tests she has scheduled. At the same time she told me that until not long ago only 3 out of 100 women were benefiting from the chemotherapy, so why take it? Especially when taking under consideration that I am stage one. The truth is that her position is based on the kind of doctor she is and the education she received. I've done some checking, she is very good in what she does and very personable, but as I have expected, she follows the conventional cancer protocol closely, without being open to any alternatives. The appointment was very educating. I have learned that my hormones work well, which is not good when diagnosed with breast cancer. Apparently cancer thrives on estrogen which in my case is positive. The cancerous cells use estrogen to grow. Her goal is to speed up my menopause to shoot down the hormone production. The pill called Tamoxifen, a type of hormonal therapy, should take care of this. She said I have to take this drug for the next 5 years.

When I was diagnosed with cancer I felt disappointingly surprised but at the same time sure that I will free myself eventually. However, when I started learning about the conventional ways of treating cancer I felt like it was the worst moment of my life, not because I was afraid of death, but because I was afraid of the treatments. The majority of people when diagnosed with cancer are terrified because it strips people physically, mentally and emotionally, leaving them just where the cancer industry wants them - vulnerable. In a vulnerable state most people will agree to do as they are told.

More people die from the treatments for cancer than of cancer itself. The treatments destroy the immune system and organs such as liver, kidneys, heart, lungs etc. People may remain alive but not in good health. I will not agree to chemo therapy, period.

Fact: Sugar feeds the cancerous cells, if we want to kill cancer we MUST eliminate sugar from our diet forever!! Instead use Stevia, which is harmless.

Question: Why have all doctors I am working with failed to tell me about the devastating effects of sugar?

About Tamoxifen: Women with estrogen receptor-positive (ER positive) breast cancer are commonly prescribed the drug tamoxifen because it blocks the effects of estrogen in breast tissue. In fact, long-term tamoxifen use among ER positive breast cancer survivors has become a standard therapy. According to the National Cancer Institute (NCI), side effects of the drug range from hot flashes, vaginal dryness, joint pain and leg cramps to blood clots, cataracts, strokes and uterine cancer. Understandably, many women are willing to accept these risks because they are told tamoxifen decreases their chance for a recurrence of breast cancer. However, a new study by Christopher Li, M.D., Ph.D., and colleagues at Fred Hutchinson Cancer Research Center just published online in the journal *Cancer Research* seems to reveal the belief that tamoxifen protects against breast cancer is only partially correct. The drug may also *cause* certain breast cancers.

Yes, breast-cancer patients who receive long-term estrogen-blocker tamoxifen therapy have a 60 percent reduction in their incidence of a second, ER positive breast cancer -- a common type of breast cancer which tends not to be aggressive and is responsive to estrogen-blocking therapy. But the new research shows tamoxifen increases the risk of the women developing a second and far more dangerous type of breast cancer by a stunning 440 percent.

March 27

Colon Hydrotherapy Appointment

I just came back from the colon hydrotherapy appointment. It went well, I feel very good, 'clean' ……………….. ☺ This was my first appointment out of a series of six. I will have two appointments each week. The Clear Path Therapies is located close to my work; I can do it at lunch.

March 28

70 Ways to Think Our Way Into Good Health

Health isn't just about exercise and eating right. The way we think and feel can have a big impact on our health as well. Here are some ways to make us happier, healthier and more fulfilled every day.

General
1. Get out negative emotions.
2. Try hypnotism.
3. Realize change is possible.
4. Think about things that energize you.
5. Imagine yourself aging more slowly.
6. Feel in control.
7. Embrace your faith.
8. Trust in yourself.
9. Be honest.
10. Live consciously.
11. Accept what comes your way.
12. Forgive yourself.

Dealing with Stress
Stress can have a big effect on physical and mental health. Here are some ways to think yourself free of it.
13. Meditate regularly.
14. Relax and let stress go.
15. Think about each breath.
16. Control your thoughts at bedtime.
17. Prepare mentally for bed.
18. Revise your dreams.
19. Concentrate on each muscle individually.
20. Allow yourself to daydream.
21. Stop worrying.
22. Set aside time to think.
23. Write in a journal.
24. Use color to control your thinking.

Illness and Disease
If you are faced with potential illness or disease here are some ways you can use the power of your brain to improve your chances of recovery.
25. Don't think about the pain.
26. Concentrate on getting better.
27. Believe in your treatments.
28. Imagine you have a strong immune system.
29. Picture your body fighting off infections.
30. Listen to your body.
31. Find a positive and friendly doctor.
32. Believe in miracles.
33. Don't fear treatments.

34. Take time to deal with negative things.
35. Stop thinking of yourself as a sick person.
36. Understand that sometimes it's all in the mind.
37. Don't expect pain.
38. Don't place blame for illness.

Emotional Health

A big part of your overall health is your happiness. Here are some ways you can boost your mental outlook just by changing your thoughts.
39. Concentrate on happiness.
40. Focus on positive aspects.
41. Start each day with optimism.
42. Smile.
43. Change your inner dialogue.
44. Reverse thoughts.
45. Give yourself compliments.
46. Use positive words in your thoughts.
47. Put positive energy out there.
48. Expect the best.
49. Think of happy memories.
50. Be friendly to yourself and others.

Diet

Help yourself stick to a healthy diet with these mental exercises.
51. Control your cravings.
52. Actively remember your last meal.
53. Concentrate on food while eating.
54. Visualize yourself as slimmer.
55. Reward yourself mentally.

Fitness

Meet your fitness goals by changing your mindset with these suggestions.
56. Think about exercise.
57. Get into the right frame of mind.
58. Think of yourself as healthy.
59. Make it a game.
60. Think of exercise as fun.
61. Envision the negative effects of your bad habits.
62. Celebrate small victories.

Personal Development
Help yourself meet your own goals and be happier and healthier overall with these mental tricks.
  63. Visualize yourself meeting goals.
  64. Downplay cynicism, ill will and envy.
  65. Remind yourself of your successes.
  66. Visualize the future.
  67. Think about what means most to you.
  68. Make your goals realistic.
  69. Fake it until you make it.
  70. Leave everything better than you found it.

March 30

Gas and Bloating
Solution

I am continuing to struggle with the bloating and gas. Majority of the time my belly is oversized making me very uncomfortable. Today I had my second colonic appointment; I was there for an hour. Brenda, my therapist, could feel the bloating and gas. She helped me tremendously, when she was done I felt wonderful, no kidding! I would recommend this treatment to anyone; everyone should cleanse periodically to stay healthy. Brenda said that it takes time for a body to adjust to eating raw vegetables. Raw fruits and veggies have their own digestive enzymes, but some are tougher than others. Some veggies are quite healthy and have both wonderful nutrients and a good amount of fiber but can cause gas and bloating:
broccoli, cauliflower, cabbage, brussels sprouts, radish, eggplant; beans and nuts are hard to break down too. Take enzymes when you eat them.

The main reason for my problem is that I have changed my diet to raw foods and my body is still getting use to it plus I might be allergic to one or two of the veggies that I eat in large amounts.

I believe that **the true solution to my problem are probiotics, enzymes, and fiber**. Even though I have written about them February 22nd, I feel that it is important I write again.

Scientific research shows 80% of our immune system lives right in our digestive tract. Based on my research, I take care of my digestive tract by taking a high quality product:

- **Probiotic**: the good bacteria, usually taken once in the morning
- **Enzymes** (Metabolic and Digestive): usually taken with each meal
- **Fiber:** cleans colon (depends on the type of fiber, once a day or with each meal)

Probiotics: they assist in digestion and improve the immune system and gastrointestinal functions. Probiotics strengthen the immune system to fight allergies, stress, exposure to toxic substances, and other diseases such as cancer.

Metabolic enzymes: responsible for energy production and detoxification. Metabolic enzymes actually facilitate our ability to think, feel, see, hear, and move. I will continue taking Wobenzymes invented by German Drs. Wolf and Benitez.

Digestive enzymes: responsible for breaking down dietary nutrients and wastes. Natural production of enzymes significantly goes down once we are 30 years old. I take the digestive enzymes with every meal.

Food enzymes: come through consumption of raw foods. Raw foods have limited enzymes, only enough to digest that particular food. I will always remember that cooking and processing destroys enzymes.

Fiber: when fiber enters the stomach, stomach acid and digestive enzymes cannot break it down. It goes to the colon. There in the colon, fiber is partially digested by the good bacteria (probiotics) allowing the good bacteria to multiply and make us healthier. Here are some of the properties that fibers have in our body:

- Stimulates peristaltic action in the colon preventing constipation

- Acts as a cleaner scraping waste off your colon walls
- Helps us lose weight by absorbing fats and toxins and preventing them from being reabsorbed.
- Move stools faster through the colon, preventing excess carbohydrates from being absorbed
- Helps us prevent colon cancer by moving toxic stools quickly out of your body

Below are few recommendations on fiber. I use Fibrezon from Amazon Herbs, http://herbswin.amazonherb.net

1. Flaxseed meal 4 tablespoons per day in water, juice, a smoothie or sprinkled on food. Recommended brands are Fiproflax by Health from the Sun, Spectrum, or Barleans. Available at Central Market, Whole Foods, Sun Harvest or People's Pharmacy
2. Organic Triple Fiber Max by Advanced Naturals. Available at Sun Harvest or Whole Foods.
3. 4 Fiber by Genesis Today. Available at Whole Foods or Central Market.
4. MetaFiber by Metagenics. At People's Pharmacy

Foods that are high in fiber include:
whole grain products, fruits and vegetables, and oatmeal.

Foods that have been proven to help the digestion process:
- organic food products
- flaxseed oil
- green tea

Foods that you may want to avoid and can effect digestion:
- synthetic sweetener
- foods coated with pesticides i.e unwashed and not organic fruit and vegetables
- alcohol
- soft drinks
- hormonally-treated products

Fact: Another way to stimulate the bowel movement is taking three glasses of water, first thing in the morning. One goes into the stomach and rest goes straight into the gut. Within half an hour, the water clears the bowel.

April 1

Budwig Protocol

Here again is my breakfast routine. I diligently have the cottage cheese and flaxseed oil mixture every morning. Flax oil mixed with sulfurated protein such as organic cottage cheese is a proven and documented cancer preventative and cure. The works of Dr. Johanna Budwig documenting the cures she performed with a bottle of flax oil and a carton of quark, a European cheese similar to cottage cheese, they are readily available from online booksellers. Johanna cured hundreds of cancer victims who had been sent home to die, and was nominated for several Nobel Prizes. Yet our traditional doctors have never heard of the Budwig protocol.

Mix four tablespoons of organic flax oil for each 100 pounds of body weight into a 1/4 to 1/2 cup of organic cottage cheese until it is bonded and no oil is left standing. What you will have then is the most proven, highly documented cancer cure and prevention on earth. It's just that simple.

This mixture of electron rich fats from flax oil with sulphurated protein from cottage cheese creates water solubility allowing electrons from the flax oil to be carried right into the cells to re-energize and oxygenate them. When cells are energized and oxygenated, cancer cannot get started and any tumors that are there melt away.

Cancer cells react to oxygenation the way a vampire would react to broad daylight: they shrivel up and die. And when healthy cells get more oxygen, they produce more energy, and our health becomes more vibrant. Basically, the Budwig protocol blasts the cancer cells with oxygen, and it also brings more oxygen to healthy cells.

Every cell in our body needs Omega 3, an essential fatty acid, both for the cell membrane and inside the cell. But the typical American does not get enough Omega 3. According to Dr. Budwig, one of the richest sources of Omega 3 is flax oil. When we take Budwig protocol, the cancer cells get an infusion of Omega 3 followed by a blast of fresh oxygen, and millions of cancer cells die on regular schedule. When we blend cottage cheese with the flax oil, not only does the cottage cheese lose its dairy properties, but also the mixture becomes water soluble. This water solubility is why the Budwig protocol delivers Omega 3 to the cells so efficiently and effectively.

Visit Budwig Center for more information regarding Budwig Protocol http://www.budwigcenter.com/johanna-budwig-biography.php

April 4

Farmer's Markets

We should provide consistent nourishment for maintaining our health. One of the best venues is either growing our own organic food or shopping in local Farmers Markets that provide high quality, fresh, and organic produce. Access to fresh, nutritious, affordable food is vital for good health and preventing disease. There are several Farmers Markets in the Austin area open to public almost every day of the week. I am sure all cities in the US have many Farmer Markets that can be found via internet.

This morning I went to Sunset Valley Market, the closest one to my house, very good experience. I purchased beautiful tomatoes, onions, lettuce, kale, and kalarepa; everything fresh, very tasty, and less expensive than organic veggies from grocery stores. There were many stands dedicated to fresh vegetables. In addition they had breads, some art and interesting landscaping plants, even some clothes. Many people came with their dogs, making the whole experience more enjoyable. Next time I will take Jazzy with me, she'll have a blast.

I am also a member of CSA (Community Supported Argiculture), I receive on bi-weekly basis share of seasonal organic vegetables, fruits, and herbs from the local farmer called Johnson's Backyard Garden. http://www.jbgorganic.com/csa/

April 7

10 Ways to Instantly Build Self Confidence

Self confidence is the difference between feeling unstoppable and feeling scared. Although many of the factors affecting self confidence are beyond our control, there are a number of things we can consciously do to build self confidence.

The bottom line is: self confidence makes us feel good, feeling good makes us happy, being happy influences our health in a very positive way.

1. Dress Sharp
When you don't look good, it changes the way you carry yourself and interact with other people. Use this to your advantage by taking care of your personal appearance. This doesn't mean you need to spend a lot on clothes. One great rule to follow is "spend twice as much, buy half as much". Rather than buying a bunch of cheap clothes, buy half as many select, high quality items.

2. Walk Faster
People with confidence walk quickly. They have places to go, people to see, and important work to do. Even if you aren't in a hurry, you can increase your self confidence by putting some pep in your step.

3. Good Posture
People with slumped shoulders and lethargic movements display a lack of self confidence. They aren't enthusiastic about what they're doing and they don't consider themselves important. By practicing good posture, you'll automatically feel more confident.

4. Personal Commercial
One of the best ways to build confidence is listening to a motivational speech. Unfortunately, opportunities to listen to a great speaker are few and far between. You can fill this need by creating a personal commercial. Write a 30-60 second speech that highlights your strengths and goals, then recite it in front of the mirror aloud whenever you need a confidence boost.

5. Gratitude
Set aside time each day to mentally list everything you have to be grateful for. Recall your past successes, unique skills, loving relationships, and positive momentum.

6. Compliment other people
When we think negatively about ourselves, we often project that feeling onto others. Get in the habit of praising other people. Refuse to engage in backstabbing gossip and make an effort to compliment those around you.

7. Sit in the front row
In schools, offices, and public assemblies around the world, people constantly strive to sit at the back of the room. By deciding to sit in the front row, you can get over this irrational fear and build your self confidence. You'll also be more visible to the important people talking from the front of the room.

8. Speak up
By making an effort to speak up at least once in every group discussion, you'll become a better public speaker, more confident in your own thoughts, and recognized as a leader by your peers.

9. Work out
Physical fitness has a huge effect on self confidence. If you're out of shape, you'll feel insecure, unattractive, and less energetic. By working out, you improve your physical appearance, energize yourself, and accomplish something positive.

10. Focus on contribution
If you stop thinking about yourself and concentrate on the contribution you're making to the rest of the world, you won't worry as much about your own flaws. The more you contribute to the world, the more you'll be rewarded with personal success and recognition.

April 8

How Our Thoughts Can Cause or Cure Cancer

Our mind can create, or CURE, disease. Our mind doesn't care which one. We can think of our body as a blank page, waiting for us to tell it what to do. Unfortunately, our body is not set to some magical "good" default so that it will automatically convert all our thoughts to a beneficial result. It is completely neutral to the outcome, and only we can control the signals.

Unfortunately, most people tend to be caught up with their negative emotions. This is an easy trap to fall into as it seems to be the cultural norm. So we may easily allow fear, anxiety, anger, sadness, guilt or countless other negative thoughts to interfere with our day. Yet, when we do this, our body will manifest these negativities into physical disease.

The placebo effect, the very real phenomenon of people becoming healed after taking a sugar pill or other sham treatment, is directly a result of our mind believing that we will get better after the fake treatment. It works both ways. The "nocebo effect" refers to the fact that, just as positive beliefs can heal us, our negative beliefs can make us sick.

What do you think would happen if everyone started to tap into their inner ability to heal disease and stopped relying on drugs and surgeries? Pharmaceutical companies would lose out big time, and so they would rather keep us completely in the dark and in fear.

Our beliefs are energy fields, and they are working to promote either health or disease in our body. Which one is up to us. When it comes to the ability of our mind to heal us, there are NO limitations. The sky is the limit. However, there is something we should remember. Other people can influence our perception of things and ultimately our ability to express the true beliefs.

I feel thrilled to have learned the information I am including in my writing; however, when I share it with some people that I know, they are not open to it. Their closed mind and negativity can easily transfer to me and cause doubt which I am not allowing to happen. This would make my mind unable to manifest healing. I am careful who I give this book to.

One more thing, cancer affects the mind, body, and spirit. A proactive and positive spirit will help me survive. Anger, unforgiveness and bitterness put the body into a stressful and acidic environment. **It is important to have a loving and forgiving spirit, to be relaxed and enjoy life.**

Positive words and affirmations are the types of thoughts we want to have floating through our mind and coming out of our mouth. In this way we reprogram our thought patterns and with it our whole life. We fill our lives with the images that we focus on. Focus on love and love will come to us; focus on the bad and we will feel bad, look bad, and our relationships will be bad. This is a simple fact of reality. To master it all, we have to do is literally change our mind.

I try to start each day with positive affirmations such as "today I will be the best and most positive I can be". Then as I go about my day, I can actually do it. I go out of my way to find the positive in every thought and situation even if I have to say that it was an "opportunity to learn" or a "challenge to be accomplished". No more doom and gloom; only a positive outlook and the positive, happy, well balanced life I want ahead of me.

April 9

How the Body Works

I want to know more about my body and how it works and here is what I have learned. Our organs are collections of specialized tissues, and our tissues are collections of groups of cells. So in reverse order, a simple, big picture looks like this:

Our cells are the basic living units that make up our body.

Groups of cells come together to form specialized tissues.

Groups of tissues come together to form our organs.

The health of every organ in our body is determined by the health of the cells that make up our organs. When the majority of cells that make up any organ in our body are healthy, that organ is likely to be healthy. Given all of the above, it makes sense, then, that taking care of our organs requires that we take care of our cells.

The most important determinant of the health of every cell in our body is the quality of blood that is supplied for ongoing nourishment and removal of waste products. The blood that our heart pumps to all of our cells delivers nutrients and oxygen to fuel ongoing energy production within our cells. So just as our heart delivers nutrients and oxygen to the cells of our kidneys, stomach, and liver, our heart also delivers nutrients and oxygen to its own cells. If the cells of our heart don't receive steady, quality blood flow, our heart will eventually lose its capacity to pump blood, nutrients, and oxygen to the rest of our body.

The main point here is this: all of the cells that make up the many organs in our body have the same basic requirements to stay healthy, with the first and most important requirement being steady blood flow. Clearly, the healthier our diet and lifestyle are, the healthier our blood will be. And the healthier our blood is, the healthier our cells will be. When we eat foods that are rich in vitamins, these nutrients touch all of our cells, not just the cells that make up our brain, bones, and teeth. In the same vein, when we expose ourselves to prescription drugs, recreational drugs, and other environmental pollutants, all of our cells are touched.

We have **eleven organ systems** that govern all of our physiological activities. They are as follows:

- **Nervous System:** director of all of our body's moment-to-moment activities.
- **Endocrine System:** same as nervous system
- **Cardiovascular System:** delivers oxygen to our cells
- **Respiratory System:** brings oxygen, maintains blood pH
- **Digestive System:** provides fuel to produce energy
- **Urinary System:** filters waste and extra fluid from your blood

- **Muscular System:** allows us to move
- **Skeletal System:** physical protection and structural support to other organ systems
- **Integumentary (Skin) System:** plays critical role in preventing infections
- **Immune System** (includes Lymphatic System): protects
- **Reproductive System**: ability to reproduce

Each of our organ systems are groups of organs that work together to carry out specific duties in our body.

Here are the main points:

1. All of our organs are influenced by all of our food and lifestyle choices. There's virtually no way to affect just one organ system via a specific diet or therapy. Whenever one of our organ systems improves or declines in health, the rest of our organ systems follow suit to some degree.
2. The health of each of our organs is determined by the health of the cells that make up our organs. And all of our cells have the same basic requirements to stay healthy.

April 10

Understanding Health

In the western countries many people see health as a black and white concept. It may be more useful to look at health as a gray scale of 1 to 100 (1 being almost dead and 100 being incredibly healthy). In this way a person can always be motivated to get healthier. As a person progresses down the scale to ill health that's when they start to have diseases that a doctor can identify like heart disease, cancer, osteoporosis, etc. These conditions could have been prevented had the person looked at health in the way of getting healthier way before they got sick.

What exactly is health?

According to the Ayurveda system (system of traditional medicine native to the Indian and practiced in other parts of the world as a form of alternative medicine), health can be seen from several different layers. At the core is spiritual health, defined as living a life in harmony with your true purpose in life. Another aspect to spiritual health is to lead a life that does not cause harm to other living beings. This is why in Ayurveda a vegetarian diet is recommended for spiritual life. Spiritual health is more important than physical health, but it is also the basis of all other forms of health such as emotional and mental health.

The next layer of health is our mental and emotional health. The Bach flower remedies were introduced because Dr. Bach recognized this level of importance. He believed that mental and emotional health imbalances usually lead to physical diseases. Nature, in her wisdom, has given people natural remedies that help restore health.

Chinese and Indian medicines also recognize the importance of this layer for optimum health. In Chinese Medicine, for example, someone who gets angry a lot can easily get liver problems. Too much sadness affects the function of the heart, etc. Herbs, acupuncture, exercise and lifestyle changes will help bring a person back into balance.

The last layer of health is physical health. If a person is spiritually and emotionally healthy then physical health is a lot easier to come by. This is the level where exercise, etc. comes into play. There are many people in the Western world who just emphasize this level of health. Bodybuilders, joggers, etc. sometimes suddenly get cancer or drop dead from a heart attack and people wonder, why? It's not a mystery. It's usually because they have been out of balance on the deepest layers of health.

Which activities should we engage in, in order to stay healthy?

On a spiritual level of health, activities such as meditation, prayer and humility help one to understand one's true purpose in life as well as to generally get more in touch with deeper aspects of the self.

Following practices of ahimsa (non violence), also enhance a person's spiritual health. Taking a caring, rather than a judgmental, attitude toward all living entities will also enhance a person's spiritual health.

Another aspect of spiritual health is service. It is the nature of the human being to serve someone other than him/herself, putting spiritual service, of some sort, as a major component in health.

April 11

Summary of my alternative cancer treatments

Since I have decided against the chemotherapy I continue research the alternative cancer treatments. The main goal they all have is to strengthen my immune system and make my cells healthy. Cancer is not as strong as most people believe it is. In fact, cancer cells are actually weak, deformed, and confused. No cancer cell has ever been known to attack a healthy cell. Cancer can not grow inside a strong, healthy body. Cancer can only thrive inside a weakened, unhealthy body. It's that simple.

Currently, in addition to vitamins, minerals, enzymes and fiber, I am also under the following protocols that are proven to kill cancer cells and boost the immune system:

- **80% Raw food** / 20% Cooked food diet, no Processed foods
- **Budwig** Flax Oil & Cottage Cheese mixture with pineapple for breakfast every morning (read April 1)
- **Beta Glucans** biological defense modifiers that nutrionally enhance, modify and balance the immune system.
- **Graviola** extract from a tree in Amazon rain forest with a strong ability to prevent abnormal cellular division, it also shrinks cancer cells without harming healthy cells. Graviola is many times stronger than

chemotherapy. In addition, it protects the immune system, fights bacterial and fungal infections, lowers high blood pressure, and is used for depression, stress and nervous disorders.

- **Green Tea Extract** cancer cells maintain telomeres which may be the secret to their immortality. Telomeres are crucial to the life of the cell, they keep the ends of the various chromosomes in the cell from accidentally becoming attached to each other. Green Tea Extract inhibits telomerase of cancer cells.
- **Vitamin C** 6000mg. An antioxidant that gets rid of free radicals which can attach to cells and damage them; immune system protector.
- **Cats Claw** is a large, woody vine that grows in Central America. Cat's claw has been used for over 2,000 years for treatment of numerous health problems and since the early 1990s as cancer treatment. Cats Claw greatly reduces inflammation, prevents blood clots and thins the blood.
- **Barley Grass** very nutritional food, a powerful antioxidant providing all nine essential amino acids which our body can not produce, builds alkalinity.

I am convinced that soon I will have detectable results of my efforts. In my constant research I discover new cancer treatment protocols that I am tempted to include together with what I am already implementing. I have decided to add two more, try them and then send urine for testing. The last time my score was 52.2 out of 100. This time if the number is less than 50, I am cancer free.

Here are two additional treatments I will start this week, once the product arrives.

- **Essiac** one of the oldest and most highly regarded alternative cancer treatments, since the 1920s thousands of cancer patients were treated successfully. Essiac is a combination of herbs.
- **Resveratrol** a member of the bioflavonoid family of fruits and vegetables inhibiting certain enzymes cancer cells use to duplicate and grow. Resveratrol is also found in the skin of red grapes and is a constituent of red wine. Several recent research studies have revealed that

resveratrol is highly effective against breast cancer by inhibiting ER positive and negative cell proliferation, cell cycle progression, and primary breast tumor growth. Resveratrol is protective of the liver even against alcohol. Be sure to look for resveratrol made from muscadine grapes that use whole grape skins and seeds, as this is where many of the benefits are concentrated.

Resveratrol is unique among antioxidants because it can cross the blood-brain barrier to help protect our brain. Other benefits include:

- o Protects cells from free radical damage
- o Lowers the blood pressure
- o Keeps heart healthy
- o Normalizes anti-inflammatory response
- o Prevents Alzheimer

I wanted to write a little more about the **Beta Glucan**, which I believe is a strong cancer fighter significantly increasing the effectives of the immune system. Beta Glucan has been subjected to rigorous studies at numerous universities, below are its features and benefits that were discovered.

Features	Benefits
Increases production of white blood cells	More immune cells can fight invaders more effectively
Increases cellular mobilization	Immune cells can respond to harmful invaders faster
Increases phagocytic capacity	Phagocytes (machrophages) can destroy more harmful invaders faster by eating them
Increases production of reactive oxygen intermediates (ROIs)	More ROIs are able to more effectively help the immune system fight a harmful invader
Helps shift the immune response from an overstimulated Th2 to a balanced Th1 response	Anecdotal evidence suggests this may help with allergies, autoimmune disease, and cancer.

April 13

Pineapple
Walnuts

Since the beginning of February every day I eat flax oil, cottage cheese, and fresh **pineapple** for breakfast. Adding pineapple to the cheese mixture was my idea, other fruits did not work for me. So I am eating pineapple for close to three months now and today I found a very interesting article in the Natural News talking about the pineapple's benefits. Here is the summary.

Bromelain, the key enzyme in pineapple, banishes inflammation as effectively as drugs. It reduces swelling, helps against sore throat, treats arthritis and gout, and speeds digestion of proteins. New research is showing pineapple to be highly effective at cancer prevention and treatment. Bromelain keeps cancers from getting started and shrinks tumors. In a study reported on March 30, in the *Cancer Letter*, scientists at the Indian Institute of Toxicology Research noted the anti-inflammatory, anti-invasive, and anti-metastatic properties of bromelain. Antioxidants in pineapple protect the immune system. Bromelain offers protection and treatment for macular degeneration.

There are several varieties of pineapple on the market. Some are ripe while still green in color, and others turn to gold when ripe. Smelling the pineapple is one way to tell it is ripe. If it gives off a sweet, fresh tropical smell, it is ready to eat. Another way to tell a ripe pineapple is to pull one of the leaves in its top knot. If the leaf remains stubbornly attached, the pineapple is not ready. The day those leaves can be easily pulled out is the day the pineapple has reached its peak of ripeness and is loaded with sweet, tangy flavor.

To prepare pineapple, cut the top off and make a narrow cut across the bottom. Place the remaining pineapple upright on a cutting board and slice off the outer skin at a depth that cuts off most of the eyes. The few eyes that remain can be eaten or cut out individually. To separate the succulent meat of the pineapple from its hard inner core, make four top-to-bottom slices around the core. This allows the pineapple to be removed from the core in four large blocks.

Healthy way to consume pineapple is Pineapple and Kale Smoothie:
1 1/2 cups cold water
Half a pineapple, cored and chopped
2 cups washed kale
Blend ingredients in blender

In the 100th Cancer Annual Meeting 2009 in Denver, Elaine Hardman, Ph.D., offered the 'eat more **walnuts**' advice based on her cancer research. The study she presented at the meeting strongly suggests the nuts can reduce the risk of breast cancer -- a disease the National Cancer Institute says took about 50,000 lives last year in the U.S.

The scientists found that when the mice ate walnuts regularly, there was a significant decrease in the incidence of breast tumors, the number of glands with a tumor and the size of tumors. Researchers found that walnuts apparently had tumor-fighting abilities. Dr. Hardman pointed out that eating walnuts may provide the body with not only essential omega-3 fatty acids, but also antioxidants and phytosterols that reduce the risk of breast cancer. In fact, there's a host of evidence suggesting that walnuts have multiple health benefits. For example, they can reduce damage to arteries and keep them flexible. And another study by Japanese researchers published recently in the *Journal of Agriculture and Food Chemistry* found that polyphenols in walnuts can prevent liver damage induced by toxic chemicals.

April 14

Poisoning foods

We can gain tremendous health benefits by omitting the "four white evils" from our diet: dairy products, refined salt, sugar and wheat, as well as other processed gluten grains. Many times it's not just what we eat that keeps us healthy, but also what we omit from our diet. These four "foods" have been so highly refined and processed that they can no longer be considered real foods. By omitting wheat, dairy, sugar and salt we also are protecting our mental and emotional health that is very negatively impacted by eating these "foods".

Refined Sugar – our body doesn't like it since it has trouble digesting and making use of it. Sugar promotes the growth of disease causing yeasts and fungi, because of fungal toxins that are found in the sugar grains. Sugar encourages our bad stomach bacteria to grow and overwhelm the digestive tract. And that's just for starters. Sugar is also acidic in nature changing the body's ph balance

Sugar in all its forms is the number one source of calories in the American diet. It is also the number one reason 66 percent of Americans are overweight, and half of that group is obese. The list of sugar consumption related health problems, over and above those associated with weight gain and obesity, is long and impressive. Conditions and diseases that affect every square inch of you, inside and out, can be directly or indirectly the result of excessive sugar intake. From problems with your eyesight to the very structure of your DNA -- from tooth decay to fluid retention to Alzheimer's to cancer -- sugar can play a role.

What to avoid:
- All artificial sweeteners, such as: NutraSweet, Equal, Splenda, sucralose and others
- The obvious sweet and dessert-type stuff -- candy, gum, cookies, cakes, pies, pastries, ice cream, etc.
- Cane syrup
- Corn syrup and corn sugar
- Invert sugar
- All the -- oses, including dextrose, fructose, glucose, lactose, and maltose

Sugar makes you old! Eating sugar causes our body to secrete high levels of insulin. Insulin and the stress hormone, cortisol, are two hormones that can dramatically speed the ageing process. Sugar depresses the immune system, it contributes to atherosclerosis, and it causes oxidative stress resulting in age spots, affecting arteries, kidneys, and brain. And the worst of all: sugar feeds cancer!

Instead of sugar, I use Stevia, Agave, or Raw Honey. These products are natural with law glycemic index, but remember, anything in excess is not good for you.

Refined Wheat – the range of processing and chemical exposure that occurs from the planting of wheat as a seed to its final processing as a grain from storage is very intense; pesticides and fertilizers, plant growing regulators which are like hormones, chemicals used in storage to protect it from critters, grain drying that is removing nutritional value, and finally the wheat processing to flour using toxic components and preservatives. Most people are not aware that even before they are planted in the ground, wheat seeds receive an application of fungicides and insecticides. Many people believe sprouted wheat bread is OK. Nothing could be further from the truth. Commercial sprouted wheat breads seem to cause the same problems as regular wheat such as celiac disease, rheumatoid arthritis, miscarriages and headaches to name a few. Intolerance to wheat is far more common than doctors typically recognize. Avoiding grains is typically wise for over 75% of the U.S. population.

White flour is also quite toxic because the healthy parts of the wheat have been removed. The lack of fiber contributes to constipation. The leaching process adds toxic chemicals to the flour and the synthetic vitamins added to replace the original ones cannot be digested. Be sure to read labels and buy breads, crackers, and cereals that contain whole grains.

I mostly use gluten free and wheat flour made out of backweat and quinoa. Go to this site for the longer list of wheat free flour: http://www.wheat-free.org/wheat-free-flour.html.

Good alternative for wheat bread is Ezekiel bread made out of grains and beans, absolutely no flour. Even though it is made with sprouted grains and has a low glycemic level this bread is soft and tasty.

Refined Salt - not all salt is created equal. There is actually a major difference between the standard, refined table and cooking salt most people are accustomed to using, and natural health-promoting salt.

Eating common table salt causes excess fluid in our body tissue, which can contribute to:
- Unsightly cellulite
- Rheumatism, arthritis, and gout
- Kidney and gall bladder stones

Salt could be the deadliest ingredient in foods, according to The Center for Science in the Public Interest (a nutritional lobbying group). They suggest that salt be regulated as a food additive to reduce its destructive presence in the food supply. Salt is a natural antibiotic so it is often used as a food preservative, but it also kills useful intestinal bacteria. Most packaged, processed foods contain excessive quantities of salt.

Ordinary table salt undergoes a great deal of processing between the factory and your grocer. This includes drying at over 1,200 degrees Fahrenheit. This high heat alters the natural chemical structure of the salt.

If we want our body to function properly, we need a balanced salt, complete with all-natural elements and free of pollutants. The important point is, today's ordinary table salt has nothing in common with natural sea salt.

The foods highest in sodium tend to be processed meats, which often contain 800 mg per 100 gram serving! At one time, salting was one of the few ways people could preserve foods. Salt kills bacteria that can cause food to spoil.

But today, between chemical preservatives and refrigeration, salt is added for other reasons — and it's added to processed foods in HUGE amounts. The reason for this has more to do with the fact that salt is an inexpensive way to improve the taste of overcooked, bland, nutrient-butchered so called food. Salt is used in high amounts in lunchmeats and cheeses to extend shelf life. Sodium also helps bind ingredients together and acts as a stabilizer.

Given that salt is absolutely essential to good health, it is important to switch to unrefined salt, an all-natural source from the Himalayas. Himalayan salt contains 84 trace minerals from our prehistoric seas, and its crystalline structure actually stores vibrational energy, which is restorative to your body.

Braggs Amino Acids can also be used for flavor and nutrients, or use lemon or lime juice or fresh herbs to enhance taste.

Pasteurized Milk - the pasteurization process, which entails heating the milk to a temperature of 145 degrees to 150 degrees F and keeping it there for at least half an hour, completely changes the structure of the milk proteins into something far less than healthy. Pasteurized cow's milk is the number one allergic food in the United States. It has been associated with a number of symptoms and illnesses including:

- Diarrhea, cramps, bloating and gas
- Osteoporosis
- Arthritis
- Heart disease
- Cancer
- Recurrent ear infections and colic in infants and children
- Type 1 diabetes
- Rheumatoid arthritis
- Infertility
- Leukemia
- Autism

The healthy alternative to pasteurized milk is raw milk, which is an outstanding source of nutrients including beneficial bacteria such as lactobacillus acidolphilus, vitamins and enzymes, and it is one of the finest sources of calcium available.

Last time I was in Barnes & Noble, I picked up a book called 'Devil in the Milk', the introduction talked about how science is indicating that a tiny protein fragment called A1 beta-casein causes a range of serious illnesses, including heart disease, type-1 diabetes, autism, and schizophrenia. Let's not forget about antibiotics and proteins that cows receive in order to produce large amounts of meat. These end up in the milk.

Fact: There is simply no more potent way to accelerate aging than sticking to a diet full of sugar and grains.

April 16

Third Breast Surgery

My third breast surgery was scheduled for Tuesday, April 14. The whole procedure was the same as before. I had to be in the hospital at 5:30am, surgery was scheduled for 7:30am. It was quick and without problems. I came back from anesthesia faster than they expected and I was ready to go home at 11:00am. This time I was in more pain than after the other two surgeries, probably because there was more breast tissue removed than before. I think my surgeon wanted to make sure that this time the margins are clear. And they are almost clear; this is what Dr. Jane said when she called this afternoon. I think to undergo radiation to make sure my breast is clear.

April 17

Appointment with Oncologist

The results from the Gene Expression Profiling Panel test came in, this test is also called Octotype DX. The report contains the Recurrence Score result, which is a number between 0 and 100. Mine was 8, this is good news.

The Ocotype DX is a unique diagnostic breast cancer test that looks at the activity of 21 different genes in a woman's breast tissue. The test measures the chance of my breast cancer returning and the likehood of my benefiting from the chemotherapy treatment. My score was low and chances of the cancer coming back are low. However, both, Dr. Jane and Dr. Beth said that the chance will be lower once I go thru the radiation and Tamoxifen.

Next steps:

- Appointment with Radiologist to learn about the radiation process
- Send urine to Philippines for testing, if the result is below 50, I will not agree to radiation. If it is above 50, I will go thru radiation.

- Meet with Dr. Beth to refuse going on 5 years Tamoxifen therapy. It apparently can reduce the chances of cancer coming back; however, the side effects, including very high possibility of another cancer, made me decide against it. I am helping myself by natural ways, which is my number one belief.
- Continue writing about my journey until I am in the recession.

April 19

Forgive – not just others, but ourselves

Forgiveness, when it becomes a way of thinking and living, is the single most powerful spiritual key to wellness. Forgiveness is a technique by which our thoughts and perceptions are changed, transforming the harmful effects of toxic emotions to the healing reality of compassion and love. Forgiveness allows us to switch our focus from fear to love; it helps us change what can be changed and allows us to make peace with the rest. This is a requirement to looking at life through spiritual eyes – a profound dimension of healing.

We hold many resentments against ourselves, we judge ourselves harshly. It is important to let go, to heal thru self-forgiveness. All of us have imperfect natures. All of us exhibit behaviors that don't match our potential. Forgiveness allows us to accept imperfection without having to approve of it.

The problem starts when we begin to judge what happened, when we label ourselves or the other person as bad, hurtful, mean, or with some other less-than-kind attribute.

The alternative? Acceptance.

Accept ourselves. Accept others. Accept that events happen. Accept that life is often far from our ideals. Forgive and accept. This is a far better way to live.
Forgive others without exception, and mean it! When we carry bitterness, hostility, and other emotional baggage, we live in the past and cannot possibly realize our potential for joy.

Because no one is perfect, forgiveness will have to be an ongoing process.

Forgive ourselves early and often, and mean it! Forgiving others might be easy. However, it's imperative to forgive ourselves, without mental reservation, for our stupid choices, inappropriate thoughts, limiting words, foolish behaviors, negative beliefs, and all the other self-defeating things we've ever done. Because we are not perfect, forgiving ourselves will be an ongoing process. We must leave the junk behind so we can make room for the joy. Practice forgiving regularly, and mean it sincerely. Acknowledge mistakes and accept forgiveness.

I try not to drag the memories of past hurts and mistakes into my present moments. Nothing from the past is important enough to allow it to pollute my present. I forgive; however, I also remember the following:

There comes a point in our life when we realize:

Who matters,
Who never did,
Who won't anymore...
And who always will.
So, don't worry about people from the past,
there's a reason why they didn't make it to the future.

April 22

Optimists Enjoy Better Health and Longevity

This relates to the power of our thoughts, the topic I have described on April 8. A large study conducted by researchers at the University of Pittsburgh School of Medicine has found that optimistic post-menopausal women were healthier and lived longer than their less upbeat counterparts. The study team had looked at data from almost 100,000 women for a period of about 8 years. The researchers defined optimism as the expectation that good things, as opposed to bad things, will take place. It was found that such women had 30% lower risk of dying from heart disease, 23% lower risk of dying from cancer. In addition, the optimists were less likely to have high blood pressure and diabetes.

There are incredibly powerful and toxic effects of negative emotions. When blood samples from people who were experiencing serious anger or fear were injected into guinea pigs, the animals dropped dead within two minutes. Now imagine what the toxins created by negative emotions such as anger, fear, frustration and stress are doing to our own bodies on a daily basis. These toxins could even be more potent health-destroyers and killers than the external poisons we ingest, inhale, and absorb every minute of every day. For people who are somewhat naturally upbeat and positive, the findings of the Pittsburgh study will come as good news. But those who tend to be a little more negative and easily discouraged should not worry, because, according to some experts, optimism is a trait that can be picked up and applied. Some useful suggestions for becoming more optimistic include staying away from negative environments, staying in the company of persons with brighter outlooks, and focusing and celebrating one's strong points instead of concentrating on the weak ones. One of the demands of living well is to no longer cling to negative emotions.

April 29

Psychic Reading

Brenda, my colon therapist, recommended that I make an appointment with her psychic. She has seen Joe a few times and each time received a reading that came out to be 90% accurate. Joe was named the "best psychic" in Austin by the Austin Chronicle's Readers' Poll. One of topics we have discussed was my breast cancer. He told me that I should continue healing by natural ways, that whatever I have chosen works and that I do not need radiation. He said radiation is a waste of money. He also said that I will be completely cured in few months, that I will live a long life. Joe said that the best is yet to come, that I am just starting my life and my fifties and sixties will be the happiest years ever. I believe it!!

So, I ask myself why cancer came to my life. To be honest, I see it as a gift. I know this sounds strange, but I don't think I would have grown in the areas that I did without this experience. Cancer was my call for personal transformation. My change is going beyond physical health habits, I am changing self-image. This is my time to replace ineffective and limited ways of living by substituting them with healthier, more effective methods, nurturing relationships and developing and pursuing my spiritual growth.

April 30

Cellular Reprogramming Statements

This exercise was given to me by a friend and I have been practicing this for over a month. I have decided to include it in my story, as part of the activities helping remove cancer from my body.

Here is what I do three times a day:

I trace the symbols shown below with my finger beginning with the figure on the right, then trace the middle figure and end with the figure on the very left. My finger stays attached to the paper, I touch the little dot in the right figure too. Then I look into a mirror and stare into the pupil of my left eye, cover my right eye with may hand, and say the following statements.

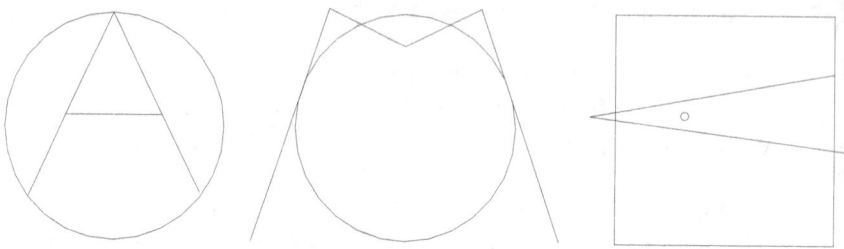

My body is healthy and whole.

My body creates only healthy cells.

I deserve a healthy body.

I enjoy my healthy body.

I trust that my body supports my healing.

This method could be applied to any health problem, I guess to any problem that we are trying to resolve. To some this might seem foolish; however, as I wrote before, believing makes things happen, which is the base of this exercise.

Here are other affirmations that I suggest:

- I am now receiving unlimited wellness.
- I love life, this is my moment.
- I am grateful for ……
- My body is producing miracles.
- I am free from worry. I know peace.
- Wellness is mine.

May 1

Relaxation and Visualization

Toxic stress is emotional overload. Toxic stress only adds to the physical and mental pain cancer brings. Stress works against wellness, putting the mind in a state of confusion, blurring the focus needed for healing. Relaxation is a simple, effective, self-healing meditation technique for reducing the effects of all kinds of stress that we live with every day. It was found that the relaxation response is even more effective when one chooses a focus word or phrase that is closely tied to one's spiritual beliefs, with significant personal meaning.

Steps on how to relax /meditate:

1. Find a quite place, free from distractions, and sit in a comfortable position.
2. Pick a focus word or short phrase that is deeply rooted in your spiritual beliefs.
3. Close your eyes and relax your muscles, from head to toe, particularly relaxing the shoulders and neck area where most tension is carried.
4. Breathe slowly and naturally. Repeat your focus word silently as you exhale.
5. Assume a passive attitude. When a distracting thought comes to mind, simply dismiss it and return to your focus word.
6. Practice this response for ten to twenty minutes twice a day.

An extension of relaxation is visualization. It is typically added at the end of the meditation period. Ongoing research leads us to believe the imagery process has an influence on the body, actually triggering a hormonal and biochemical response to a renewed sense of hope. The resulting changes to the body's chemistry influence immune function, assisting the body in maximizing its opportunity to heal.

Try this:

1. Picture your cancer cells as weak and confused.
2. Create a mental image of your treatment and your immune system overcoming the cancer.
3. Imagine your body's natural process eliminating the disease from your system.
4. Envision the cancer shrinking until it disappears.
5. Imagine yourself well, filled with vitality for living.

May 3

Guacamole Delivers Concentrated Nutrition
Salsa and Guacamole Recipe

Guacamole is good for us. While avocado has a bad reputation as being high in fat, the truth is that it ranks among the healthiest types of vegetable oil. Also, the other ingredients in Guacamole are highly alkalizing, loaded with phytonutrients and feature over 100 known health benefits. It is essential to make Guacamole fresh however as the many premade mixes (often what restaurants serve) contain no real Avocado!

Guacamole Ingredients

Tomato
Tomato contains Lycophene, a powerful antioxidant and phytonutrient, contains vitamins A, C and K along with Niacin and Calcium, helps purify the blood and improves skin clarity while reducing cholesterol and gallstones, relieves liver congestion and promotes a healthy cardiovascular system, has unique benefits in raw versus cooked form. Tomato has antiseptic properties.

Pepper
Pepper contains the antioxidant Capsaicin, an alkaloid that is some can relieve allergies and reduces pain. Peppers help treat ulcers, headaches and congestion and also reduce cholesterol, blood clotting and strokes. While, increasing metabolism Peppers also have antibacterial properties.

Garlic
Garlic contains the antioxidant Allicin, which is formed from alliin and allinase when the cloves are crushed. Garlic helps lower blood pressure and cholesterol while cleansing the liver. Offering unique health benefits when consumed in raw versus cooked or aged, garlic kills parasites and has antiviral, antibacterial, antimicrobial and antifungal properties.

Onion
Onion contains the antioxidant Quercetin along with vitamin C, vitamin E, Potassium and Folic Acid. Onion relieves allergy symptoms and congestion along with helping reduce cholesterol.

Onion can treat and prevent cataracts, atherosclerosis and coronary heart disease and helps remove heavy metals from the body. Onion has antimicrobial properties.

Cilantro
Cilantro contains several antioxidants including camphor, carvone, elemol, geraniol and limonene. A natural deodorizer, Cilantro relieves nausea, indigestion and bloating along with urinary tract infections. Consuming cilantro (whose seeds are called Coriander) helps reduce cholesterol and blood suga levels. Cilantro kills Salmonella and removes heavy metals such as Mercury from the body. Cilantro has anti-inflammatory and antibacterial properties.

Cumin
Cumin is available in both seed and powder form and contains Iron. A powerful antioxidant, Cumin helps improve digestion, strengthens the immune system and has antibacterial properties. Cumin is one of the primary flavors in many Ethnic cuisines, especially Mexican.

Lemon Juice
Fresh lemon juice contains vitamin C and has an alkalizing effect on the system. Lemon relieves stomach discomfort and removes gallstones when combined with olive oil. Lemons help prevent osteoarthritis, atherosclerosis, diabetes and kidney stones. Lemon has antibacterial, antiseptic, and antimicrobial properties. Read September 26 for more about lemons.

Apple Cider Vinegar
Raw, unfiltered apple cider vinegar contains an enzyme chain long regarded as a cure-all called Mother. Taken by Hippocrates himself, Apple cider vinegar helps relieve gout, acid reflux and arthritis. Apple cider vinegar helps reduce cholesterol, calcium deposits, allergies, acne and even muscle fatigue. Cider vinegar improves stamina and metabolism, soothes a sore throat and strengthens the immune system. Cider vinegar is also a powerful cleaning agent and kills fleas while being safe for pets.

Olive Oil
Olive Oil contains oleic acid, a healthy, monounsaturated fatty acid. Olive oil is found in the Mediterranean diet and helps reduce blood pressure, asthma and arthritis. Olive oil helps

prevent and treat diabetes and increases metabolism. Choose extra virgin oil as "pure" is normally processed with solvents including Hexane.

Avocado
Avocado contains Lutein, a carotenoid along with vitamin E, monounsaturated fat and Magnesium. Avocado helps improve the absorption of the nutrients from other foods and improves skin tone and clarity.

Lime Juice
Lime juice contains potassium and helps purify the blood and liver. Lime juice strengthens the immune system and also has antibacterial, antimicrobial and antiseptic properties.

Sea Salt
Sea salt contains many trace minerals, especially gray and pink salt. Sea salt stabilizes the heartbeat and blood sugar levels while helping the body to generate hydroelectric energy. Sea salt improves absorption and nerve cell communication while relieving the lungs and sinuses.

Salsa Recipe
The following salsa mixture is a prerequisite for Guacamole and can be used in many other recipes or enjoyed straight.

Ingredients
    4 heirloom tomatoes
    2 peppers
    2 garlic cloves
    1 onion
    1/2 cup fresh cilantro
    1 Tbsp apple cider vinegar
    1 Tbsp olive oil
    1 Tbsp lemon juice
    1 tsp cumin
Preparation
Using mortar and pestle, mash garlic, cilantro and, cumin
Add olive oil, lemon and vinegar
Dice tomato, pepper and onion
Blend ingredients together with potato masher

Guacamole Recipe

Next, simply stir salsa with fresh avocado, lime and sea salt for fast guacamole. Mixing the other ingredients together independently is something most restaurants miss (especially those serving "table side" Guacamole). Instead they serve diced vegetables suspended in Avocado. Be careful not to over-mix (green and red make brown). Storing the Avocado seeds in the mixture keeps the guacamole green longer. Refrigerate and consume within 24 hours.

Ingredients
    4 ripe avocados
    1/4 cup salsa
    1 Tbsp lime juice
    1/2 tsp Himalayan sea salt
Preparation
    Stir together avocado and salsa
    Add lime juice and salt

Other Serving Suggestions: Substitute mango for avocado for fast mango salsa (or try peach, banana or blueberry). Fresh salsa can be mixed with beans to make fast chili, tomato puree to make fast pasta sauce, black beans to make fast nacho dip, and buckwheat for a fast vegetarian meal. Salsa and buckwheat is what I eat often.

May 6

Cancer and Mushrooms, Asparagus, Papaya

Mushrooms: The result of the new study about breast cancer is that women who eat a third of an ounce of fresh mushrooms every day could decrease their chances of developing breast cancer by 64 percent! This study comes from China. China became known as the birthplace of natural cures. In fact, this study found that the daily dose of mushrooms combined with regular consumption of green tea yielded risk decrease of 90 percent. This is not the first time scientists have found evidence of mushrooms' cancer-fighting properties. Laboratory studies have found that mushrooms may suppress the body's production of the sex hormone estrogen, much like the breast cancer drugs known as aromatose inhibitors. High estrogen levels are a well-known risk factor for breast cancer.

Use Button Mushrooms, they are smaller and tend to be freshest and are most likely to feature the closed cap. A closed cap means that you can't see the tiny black fibers inside the mushroom when you turn it upside down. Avoid open cap button mushrooms as these are of inferior quality. Remember to eat organic mushrooms only!

Most mushrooms contain beta-glucan that increase DNA and RNA in the bone marrow where immune cells are made. I take beta-glucan every morning since I went on the natural protocol. In addition, I include mushrooms in my meals. In order to get the nutritional value of mushrooms they should be cooked. The cell wall of mushrooms cannot be digested unless they are tenderized by heat. Shiitake are mushrooms I eat the most.

Asparagus: Cancer might disappear as the result of using asparagus remedy. For the treatment asparagus should be cooked before using.

Procedure:
1. Place the cooked asparagus in a blender and liquefy to make a puree, and store in the refrigerator.
2. Eat 4 full tablespoons twice daily, morning and evening.

Asparagus contains a good supply of protein called histones, which are believed to be active in controlling cell growth. That accounts for its action on cancer acting as a general body tonic. In any event, regardless of theory, asparagus used as suggested, is a harmless substance.

It has been reported by the US National Cancer Institute, that asparagus is the highest tested food containing glutathione, which is considered one of the body's most potent anticarcinogens and antioxidants.

Papaya: Papaya promotes digestive health and intestinal cleansing, fights inflammation, and supports the immune system. It protects lung and joint health, revitalizes the body, and boosts energy levels. Papaya is a potent cancer fighter that is highly effective against hormone related cancers as well as

92

other cancers. New research shows papaya can stop the growth of breast cancer cells, halt metastasis, and normalize the cell cycle. The intense orangey-pink color of papaya means it is chock full of cancer fighting carotenoids. Not only beta carotene, but lycopene is found in abundance. The construction of lycopene makes it highly reactive toward oxygen and free radicals. Isothiocyanates found in papaya restore the cell cycle to eliminate cancer. Enzymes from papaya digest proteins including those that protect tumors. Eating papaya after a meal promotes digestion, and helps prevent bloating, gas production, and indigestion. Go to the end of this book for a good papaya recipe.

May 11

Urine Test Results (Second)

I have not so good news. I received my test results from Philippines; my HCG is 53 out of 100, which is 0.8 higher than the test done before my three surgeries. I found out that each surgery disturbed the cancerous cells worsening the situation. The natural ways of healing are improving my immune system and by now my cancer should be gone; however, I have agreed to three surgeries and now I have to go thru radiation. If I knew then what I know now, I would think twice about the surgery. Despite all this, I am very positive and sure that I'll get where I am going, with a small delay.

May 12

Breast Cancer Causes - 5 Reasons Why We Have Breast Cancer

There are very specific reasons why we have breast cancer. Each of these reasons is reversible. The power lies within us to get our body back to a state of balance so it can heal itself.

1) Toxins – We are all exposed to them to some degree on a daily basis. If we smoke or drink a lot of alcohol, our exposure is even higher. And if we don't have some method of detoxification and all those toxins we take in have no way to escape, they'll just settle into the tissues of our body. Remember to detox; go to July 7th for simple ways.

2) Nutritional Deficiencies - Our body is a machine. Like any other machine, it needs certain types of fuel to run at peak performance levels.

3) Electromagnetic Fields - Living near high voltage power lines, excessive computer use, cell phones. They can cause chaos and even contribute to breast cancer when levels are too high. I have attached to my cell phone a chip that protects me. Go to: http://www.thecellphonechipstore.com for more details.

4) Stress - Stress is bad news for any type of cancer, and it can definitely be a reason why we have breast cancer. So many women seem to just keep it all in with no real outlet. Dealing with stress is key if you ever want optimum health. Many days in this book are dedicated to controlling stress.

5) Personal Care Products - Many of the ingredients in most of the make-ups and skin creams women use regularly are cancer causing. A lot of them mimic estrogen in the body, which will directly lead to breast cancer. If you want to get rid of breast cancer, use only natural care products. Go to May 17 for more details.

Plus two very obvious reasons:

6) obesity vs. whole food diet, and 7) no exercise.

Wearing the right bra
While writing about the significance of personal products, I thought it would be a good time to address bras that we are wearing. In 1991 study published by the European Journal of Cancer revealed that premenopausal women who did not wear bras had half the risk of breast cancer compared with bra users. Another group of Japanese researchers discovered that wearing a girdle or bra can lower our levels of melatonin by 60%. The hormone melatonin is intimately involved with the regulation of our sleep cycles, and numerous studies have shown that

melatonin has anti-cancer activities. Simply replacing metal underwires with plastic ones is the best alternative solution if we don't want to forego the underwire entirely. Wearing metal on our body is something we generally want to avoid.

If we follow each of these suggestions we'll find that our body will begin to restore itself back to its original state of health. Breast cancer can be very difficult to deal with, but it can be overcome. <u>All you have to do is take action.</u>

May 14

Preparing for Radiation

I am starting radiation May 19th. The high doses of radiation will kill cancer cells and stop them from spreading. Cancer cells will not die right away, it takes weeks before they start to die. My treatment will last for 8 weeks, I will be going to Texas Oncology every day except for weekends. Today I had a CAT scan needed to prepare me for the treatment. I was asked to undress and lay down my upper body on a flexible material that when pumped had created a solid form around my body. This form will keep me in exactly the same position every time a high-energy beam is directed at my breast. The most common side effects are: skin changes, cough and shortness of breath, dry or sore throat, fatigue, and diarrhea. Since I am in good health besides cancer, the side affect should be very mild.

When I was waiting, I was shocked to see a big jar of chocolates and candies at each nurse station. Sugar is the worse thing for cancer patients, it feeds the cancerous cells. <u>How ignorant!</u> I couldn't disregard this once I saw a cancer patient reaching for the candy. I found Dr. Catherine's main nurse. I asked her first not to take me wrong and then I said that in many books and publications written by well establish doctors it is clearly said that sugar feeds cancer. I asked why the sugar is available in the cancer therapy center. She became very defensive and said that my information is wrong, that sugar helps cancer, and this is why they have it here. I didn't know what else to say, I didn't want to start an argument in a room full of ill people, I walked away. I was not able to help those who come there for their treatment, but hopefully my book will make a difference in other people's lives.

The theory that **sugar feeds cancer** was born nearly 80 years ago. In 1931 the Nobel Prize was awarded to German researcher Dr. Otto Warburg, who first discovered that cancer cells have a fundamentally different energy metabolism compared to healthy cells. Sugar creates an acidic pH in cancerous cells allowing them to grow.

We can starve cancer by eating foods that prevent too many blood vessels. A tumor actually needs blood in order to grow; this is how it feeds on the glucose (sugar) in our bloodstream. But angiogenesis appears to be preventable by consuming foods that are natural inhibitors of excessive blood vessel growth. When we regularly consume foods listed below, we can effectively starve any microscopic cancerous growths, effectively preventing them from growing further and becoming dangerous.

According to Dr. Li, who is currently leading this research, resveratrol from red grapes, for example, have been shown to inhibit abnormal angiogenesis by 60 %. Even more potent is the ellagic acid found in strawberries.

Other potent anti-angiogenetic foods include:
- Green Tea
- Berries
- Cherries
- Citrus: oranges, grapefruits, lemons
- Kale
- Turmeric
- Nutmeg
- Artichokes
- Parsley
- Garlic
- Tomato
- Maitake mushroom

Logically, different foods contain different potencies of anti-angiogenetic compounds. Some foods have even been found to be more potent than current anti-angiogenetic drugs! These include parsley and garlic.

May 15

Inspiring Quotes

During my first visit to the radiology center I received a calendar to monitor my treatment schedule, and in it I found few inspiring quotes. Below are couple of quotes from the Oncology Calendar plus more I found elsewhere:

" It is our choices…..that show what we truly are, far more than our abilities"
- J.K. Rowling

"Ability is what you are capable of doing. Motivation determines what you do. Attitude determines how well you do it"
- Lou Holtz

"Fools live to regret their words, wise men to regret their silence"
- Will Henry

"I have found that if you love life, life will love you back"
- Arthur Rubinstein

"The secret to living an exceptional life tomorrow is purely a matter of thinking strong, joyful thoughts today"
- Tommy Newbery

"Yesterday is history
Tomorrow is mystery ………. Today is a gift"
- Eleanor Roosevelt

"Everything will be okay in the end. If it's not okay, it's not the end. - Unknown

"Life is not about how to survive the storm; it's about how to dance in the rain"

"If you are distressed by anything external, the pain is not due to the thing itself but to your own estimate of it; and this you have the power to revoke at any moment"
- Marcus Aurelius

"When the power of love overcomes the love of power the world will know peace"
- Jimi Henfrix

"To get the full value of joy you must have somebody to divide it with"
- Mark Twain

"The good life is inspired by love and guided by knowledge"
- Bertrand Russell

"When one door of happiness closes, another opens; but often we look so long at the closed door that we do not see the one which has been opened for us."
- Helen Keller

"A man should always consider how much he has more than he wants, and how much more unhappy he might be than he really is."
- Joseph Addison

"The will of man is his happiness."
- Friedrich von Schiller

'Anger is only one letter short of danger.'
- Eleanor Roosevelt

'Life is a constant change; if you stop changing you'll stop living"

'Choose being kind over being right and you'll be right every time.' - Richard Carlson

"We are formed and molded by our thoughts. Those whose minds are shaped by selfless thoughts give joy when they speak or act. Joy follows them like a shadow that never leaves them"
- Buddha

"All destiny begins with thinking"
- Percival

"You are today where your thoughts have brought you; you will be tomorrow where your thoughts take you"
– James Allen

"Enough is as good as a feast"
- John Heywood

"May your live all the days of your life" - Jonathan Swift

"There is no happiness where there is no wisdom"
- Sophocles

"Science is organized knowledge. Wisdom is organized life."
- Immanuel Kant

"The greatest grieves are those we cause ourselves."
- Sophocles

"Our greatest glory is not in never falling, but in getting up every time we do."
- Confucius

"Before you embark on a journey of revenge, dig two graves."
- Confucius

"The first step to getting the things you want out of life is this: Decide what you want." - Ben Stein

"Life shrinks or expands in proportion to one's courage." - Anais Nin

"Everything has its beauty but not everyone sees it." - Confucius

"A friend is one who knows us, but loves us anyway"
- Jerome Cummings

May 16

Vitamin B12

Vitamin B12 is known as the energy vitamin, and our body requires it for a number of vital functions. Among them: energy production, blood formation, DNA synthesis, and myelin formation. Myelin is insulation that protects our nerve endings and allows them to communicate with one another. The older we get the more likely we are to have a vitamin B12 deficiency. The two ways we become deficient are through a lack of vitamin B12 in our diet, or through our inability to absorb it from the food we eat.

Vitamin B12 is found almost exclusively in animal tissues, including foods like beef and beef liver, lamb, snapper, venison, salmon, shrimp, scallops, poultry and eggs. However, one of the best sources, given how beef and pork is affected by today's food industry, is wild fish, organic chicken, and free-ranged organic eggs. Eggs are one of the healthiest foods in the world.

Our body needs B12 vitamin for:
- proper digestion, food absorption, iron use, carbohydrate and fat metabolism
- healthy nervous system function
- promotion of normal nerve growth and development
- help with regulation of the formation of red blood cells
- cell formation and longevity
- proper circulation
- adrenal hormone production
- healthy immune system function
- support of female reproductive health and pregnancy
- feelings of well-being and mood regulation
- mental clarity, concentration, memory function
- physical, emotional and mental energy

Symptoms of Vitamin B12 deficiency:
- mental fogginess
- problems with your memory
- mood swings, depression
- lack of motivation
- feelings of apathy

- fatigue and a lack energy
- muscle weakness
- tingling in your extremities
- it is linked to Alzheimer
- anemia
- sleep problems
- cancer

Some studies showed that it required up to 9000 micrograms per day (9mg) in order to achieve the maximum feeling of well-being. The vast majority of these studies also showed that almost no one had any ill effects from such high doses, so it's undeniable that this vitamin is safe in doses much higher than the 'standard' 1000 micrograms per day.

Interesting: vitamin B creates a body smell that keeps mosquito away, of course if we have enough of the vitamin B in our body. I spend many hours in my garden and no longer have as many mesquite bites as before.

May 17

Skin Care and Our Health
Ingredients to Avoid

Quality skin care is part of our entire package of wellbeing. Our skin grows from inside out and absorbs everything we put on it; I rarely put anything on my skin that I wouldn't be willing to put in my mouth.

Skin functions as an organ that can absorb and leak both nutrients and toxins through its pores. The condition of our skin is a powerful reflection of just how healthy we are on the inside. Because our skin has the ability to absorb whatever we put on it, careful choices are critical. We want to give our skin the same thoughtful care we give our internal organs. Let's take a quick look at some of the ingredients in today's skin care products that can compromise the health of our skin or even our body functions.

Here are a few of the most common dangerous ingredients:

- **Mineral Oil, Paraffin, and Petrolatum** -- Petroleum products that coat the skin like plastic, clogging pores and creating a build-up of toxins, which in turn accumulate and can lead to skin issues. Slows cellular development, which can cause you to show earlier signs of aging. Suspected cause of cancer. Disruptive of hormonal activity. By the way, when there's an oil spill in the ocean, don't they rush to clean it up -- fast? Why put that stuff on your skin?

- **Parabens** -- Widely used as preservatives in the cosmetic industry (including moisturizers). An estimated 13,200 cosmetic and skin care products contain parabens. Studies implicate their connection with cancer. They have hormone-disrupting qualities -- mimicking estrogen -- and interfere with the body's endocrine system.

- **Phenol carbolic acid** -- Found in many lotions and skin creams. Can cause circulatory collapse, paralysis, convulsions, coma and even death from respiratory failure.

- **Propylene glycol** -- Used as a moisturizer in cosmetics and as a carrier in fragrance oils. Shown to cause dermatitis, kidney or liver abnormalities, and may inhibit skin cell growth or cause skin irritation.

- **Acrylamide** -- Found in many hand and face creams. Linked to mammary tumors in lab research.

- **Sodium laurel** or lauryl sulfate (SLS), also known as sodium laureth sulfate (SLES) -- Found in car washes, engine degreasers, garage floor cleaners... and in over 90% of personal care products! SLS breaks down the skin's moisture barrier, easily penetrates the skin, and allows other chemicals to easily penetrate. Combined with other chemicals, SLS becomes a "nitrosamine", a potent class of carcinogen. It can also cause hair loss. SLES is sometimes disguised with the labeling "comes from coconut" or "coconut-derived".

- **Toluene** -- Poison! Danger! Harmful or fatal if swallowed! Harmful if inhaled or absorbed through the skin. Made from petroleum or coal tar, and found in most synthetic fragrances. Chronic exposure linked to anemia, lowered blood cell count, liver or kidney damage, and may affect a developing fetus. Butylated hydroxytoluene (BHT) contains toluene. Other names may include benzoic and benzyl.

- **Dioxane** -- Found in compounds known as PEG, Polysorbates, Laureth, ethoxylated alcohols. Common in a wide range of personal care products. The compounds are usually contaminated with high concentrations of highly volatile 1,4-dioxane, easily absorbed through the skin. Dioxane's carcinogenicity was first reported in 1965 and later confirmed in studies including one from the National Cancer Institute in 1978. Nasal passages and liver are the most vulnerable. Dioxane is easily removed during the manufacturing process by "vacuum stripping". Warning: It is a synthetic derivative of coconut. Watch for hidden language on labels, such as "comes from coconut".

I have used these guidelines to check the products I currently use and the products that I am planning to buy. My consciousness is clean; I do my best to take care of my skin. I suggest you do the same.

Is smooth skin a hopeless goal? Not really. These five strategies can help...

1. Hydrate your entire system with lots of water and high anti-oxidant green tea. During winter there's a tendency not to drink as much due to cool temperatures. You may want to bring your water to room temperature to encourage drinking more. Or enjoy more warm green tea.

2. Eat a healthy diet of mostly raw foods, and foods high in omega-3 fatty acids which produce a hydrating effect from the inside out.

3. Take a revitalizing bath – in warm water, not hot!
    Himalayan salt baths are rejuvenating, and help dry skin
    to slough off. Hot water is damaging to your skin, so
    stick with warm water.

4. Moisturize daily with non-clogging organic moisturizers
    such as coconut oil or body butter. These nourish your
    skin instead of clogging it, as many toxin-impaired
    moisturizers do.

5. It's especially important to cleanse and moisturize
    before you go to bed at night, to remove impurities from
    your skin before your revitalizing sleep time. Just be
    sure your moisturizer isn't tainted with toxins.

May 21

Typical radiation visit

Today is the third day of radiation, the routine is settled, it will
be the same till middle of July, if I do not miss any days. I have
to be there every day but weekends. On Wednesdays, after
radiation, I meet with Dr. Catherine for the status update,
including answers to my questions, checking my vital signs, and
observing changes happening to my body.

I leave work 20 minutes before my appointment; the Oncology
Center is not too far. Upon arrival I sign in at the reception
desk and wait for the radiation technician to call my name. I go
to the changing room where I remove all my clothes from waist
up and put the hospital gown on. I sit down on a chair across
from the radiation room and wait for my turn. The radiation
room is large, with dimmed light, quiet music, and very large
radiation therapy equipment in the middle of it. I lay down on a
table with my upper body inside the form which was created
just for me during my first visit. There are three big marks on
my belly, just under both breast, and one large mark on my
right breast, where the tumor use to be. These marks will stay
with me thru the entire radiation. There are red laser beams
shooting down from the hole in the ceiling. My feet are tied with
a belt, my body is in the form, I am not allowed to move. Two

technicians move me to make sure that the body marks are exactly under the red laser beams. Once they are happy with my position they leave the room and the radiation begins. A huge arm moves around me stopping three times. Every time it stops the high-energy radiation beam penetrates my breast. I do not feel much, maybe a little warmth. The technician comes back to the room, lets me off the table. I go back to the changing room, place healing ointment on my breast, then dress and leave.

May 23

Stay Connected

Research shows that friendships not only enhance our life but also protect and improve our health. And studies show that the happiest people are those who have both good mental health and good social relationships.

The relationships we have with people outside our family — our friends, co-workers, neighbors, and others we have daily contact with. Whom do we consider our friends? Would we like closer relationships with them, or to spend more time with them?

Friendships take time and tending the same way that our relationships with our family do, and it's natural to put our jobs and families ahead of our friends. But making time for people whom we connect with and can laugh with enriches our life. Keeping in touch — whether by phone, e-mail, letters, or get-togethers — is an essential part of staying close. Today's small change is to reconnect with a friend, perhaps someone we haven't seen or spoken to in longer than we had intended. Chances are good that our friend misses us too, and will be delighted that we took the initiative to catch up. This is what happened to me, now my life has another soul in it that cares and helps me go thru my cancer experiences.

Sometimes friends grow apart; as new friendships are made through circumstance or shared interests, others are lost. It may be that with an old friend we don't have much in common anymore, or have too much going on in our lives to stay meaningfully connected. But if it is a relationship that's really important to us, we may want to talk to our friend about our relationship before we drift apart for good. Tell the friend how you feel and ask if there's a way to reconnect. There may also be something going on in their life that has affected them — something we don't know about. We won't know unless we ask.

May 24

Cancer is not a Disease

Today I read about the theory that a person grows cancer cells in order to keep them from dying of the real causes of illness. In truth, **cancer is on our side, not against us.** Cancer is part of the body's complex survival responses and not a disease. It appears to be a highly confusing and unpredictable disorder. It can strike anyone at any time. But when truly looking at the reasons behind the development of cancer cells, it appears that cancer is not as coincidental or unpredictable as it seems to be.

Cancer, the physical disease, generally occurs when there is a strong undercurrent of emotional uneasiness and deep-seated frustration. Cancer does not cause a person to be sick; it is the sickness of the person that causes the cancer. Successfully treating cancer requires the patient to become whole again on all levels of the body, mind and spirit.

Cancer can have no power or control over us, unless we allow it to grow in response to the beliefs, perceptions, attitudes, thoughts, and feelings we have, as well as the life choices we make. Yet in truth, most cancers appear and disappear of their own accord. Not a day passes without the body making millions of cancer cells. Some people, under severe temporary stress, make more cancer cells than usual and form clusters of cancerous cells that disappear again once they feel better. The problem is that people who are diagnosed are terrified and they submit their bodies to these cutting/burning/poisoning procedures that cause more harm.

Extensive scientific research over the past 10 years has proved that genes do not cause disease, but are, in fact, influenced and altered by changes in the environment throughout life. The possibility that **cancer is a survival mechanism** has never been considered in cancer treatments, and this has fatal consequences. For many cancer patients whose immune systems are already compromised, just one dose of chemotherapy or radiation can turn out to be fatal.

Cancer cells are healthy cells that have mutated genetically so that they can live in an environment where oxygen is not available. When cells are deprived of vital oxygen (their primary source of energy), some of them will die, but others will manage to alter their genetic software program and mutate in a most ingenious way so that they can live without oxygen.

Cancer is not a disease; it is the final and most desperate survival mechanism the body has. It only takes control of the body when all other measures of self-preservation have failed. Healing is accepting, allowing and supporting, not fighting or resisting. There is something to be learned from every situation, including having cancer. A person's willingness to face, accept and learn from the issues that cancer changes into a purposeful, potentially uplifting and sometimes even euphoric experience. This is how I feel most of the times, better than before.

Our presence in the body and what we do, eat, drink, feel and think determine how well our genes are able to control and sustain our physical existence. Disease is a provider of new life. Cancer only strikes when a part or parts of us are not alive anymore, physically, emotionally, and spiritually. Cancer can actually be viewed as a way out of a deadlocked situation that paralyzes the heart of a person, it helps to break down old, rigid patterns.

Furthermore, we need to love every cell in our body, including the cancer cells if we want to live in health and peace. Cutting them out of the body through surgery or destroying them with poisonous drugs or deadly radiation adds even more violence to the body than it already has to deal with.

To help someone who is going through the disease process, allow them to experience the pain, despair, confusion, loneliness, hopelessness, anger, fear, guilt, and shame that they have been suppressing. If the afflicted person knows that he or she can have all these feelings without having to hide them, cancer can become a very powerful means of self-healing.

Cells only go into a defensive mode and turn malignant if they need to ensure their own survival, at least for as long as they can. A spontaneous remission occurs when cells no longer need to defend themselves. Cancer is the final attempt of the body to live, and not, as most people assume, to die.

Cancer growth usually occurs in areas of severe dehydration. The cells can run dry for a number of reasons:
- Lack of water intake
- Consumption of beverages that have diuretic effects like coffee, caffeinated tea, soda pop, and alcohol.
- Consumption of stimulating foods or substances, such as meat, hot spices, sugar and tobacco.
- Stress
- Most pharmacological drugs
- Excessive exercise
- Overeating and excessive weight gain
- Watching television daily for several hours

If you have cancer, also avoid:
- Chlorinated water
- Fluoride in municipal drinking water
- Wireless devices
- Pesticides and other chemical toxins
- Hair dye
- Arsenic, asbestos, and nickel
- Teflon
- PVC shower-curtains
- Artificial sweeteners such as Aspartame and Splenda
- Growth hormones in cows milk
- Synthetic vitamins
- Grilling meat, poultry or fish
- High intake of fructose and sucrose
- Smoking cigarettes
- Sunscreens
- Night Shift Work
- Blood transfusions

If we find the purpose and meaning in the occurrence of a cancer we will also find the way to cure it. Tracing a cancer back to its origins is the key to true healing. Cleansing, pampering and nourishing the body are acts of accepting responsibility for what is happening to us and we become in control of our body and life.

May 28

Not so Good Day - Fear
And Some Good News

Last night I was very uncomfortable, my breast was hot, swollen, and sore. Every time I moved, I felt pain. This is the first time I have noticed the affects of radiation. In the morning I made a decision to take a break.

I decided to go to the oncology center, but only to deny the therapy for today. My mind was made up! At least this is what I thought. Once they heard me, I was taken to a room I had not seen before. The radiation technician started convincing me to change my mind. I realized that everything she was saying she had said before to somebody else who was in the same situation as mine. She was manipulating me to go through the treatment, no matter what I was saying or how strong I was, she was winning. Once I gave in I started to cry. Not because I was going to go through the radiation but because I agreed to something I did not want to do. I was not forced to do it, I was convinced to do something against my will by injecting fear to my mind. I lost! I cried through the whole procedure. In the end I apologized for showing weakness. They understood. I am sure they have witnessed this before.

Fear is very powerful! I have experienced the medical society power. I gave in easily because this is what most of us do for so long without question. You might say that what they did was assistance, but not when it was not what I wanted to do.

Information is power changing each of us and making us responsible for our own lives. I have noticed that if something is right for me, my decision to do it is not fear based ... except when it comes to cancer treatment. I believe now that doctors and medical staff are using fear to convince us of therapies our bodies may not be in harmony with.

Except for what I have experienced today, I feel good. The supplements that I am taking are making big difference; I am full of energy and optimism. My mind is clear, I understand why I have cancer and I am eliminating behaviors and situations that might have caused it. I am very devoted to my diet and I exercise on regular basis. I am now concentrating on my mind and how to better control it. Many of my writing days were and will be dedicated to techniques that help eliminate the negative emotions. I am practicing what I have learned and I am reading more about the abilities of my mind to heal me. In few days I will write about this interesting book I am currently reading. It describes another helpful approach to become as happy and free as I can be.

The company that I work for organizes a health screening each year. Here are the results from the screening done few days ago:

Triglycerides: 79 (range units 0-149)
Total cholesterol: 157 (range units 100-200)
Chol/HDL Ration: 2.7 (range units 0-4.4)
HDL Cholesterol: 59 (range units >39)
LDL: 82 (range units 0-100)

The 2009 results are better than 2007 and 2008. I am improving my health significantly. It is obvious that changes I have introduced to my life are making big difference.

My Cancer Prevention Score improved 9.1% since last year and it is above the National Average – HOW IRONIC. Last year I was at 61.7% compared with 70.8%, the National Average is 68.4%. This proves that cancer is in our body for a long time before they become large enough to see with the existing methods of testing.

My Total Health Power Score has increased 10.2% since my last year screening. Today it is 74.4%, 6.8% above the National Average. This is very good news!

May 31

Random Thoughts

It is important to remember that cancer is a different kind of illness that demands a different kind of response, it demands our participation. Wellness is not an accident, it requires effort. What is personally contributed to recovery makes a significant difference.

My faith is that my immune system will become strong enough that I can rejoin the rest of the world soon, but at the same time stick to what I have learned as an important way of living. The beauty of true healing is that eventually it creates health. In regards to eating, the food becomes like a checking account, I can take a vacation if I make regular deposits. Once in a while I'll have pizza or a good burger …. yummy.

Another important thought; **life comes down to the choices we make, and then living with the results.** It's important to remember that we almost always have options – healthier options. Some require more work than others, but in this case it really will not take much to make a meaningful change that can help us have a healthier body and life.

It is important to take time to understand that cancer can be completely cured by building up the body, not by tearing it down.

June 1

Managing Stress

Stress can have a huge impact on every aspect of our life, so stress reduction is necessary for maintaining both our physical and emotional health. Since we can't simply wish stress away, managing stress is a vital skill to develop.

Certain situations create stress instantly, such as when there's an urgent problem that requires our immediate attention. Managing stress is important so that we can think clearly. Here are some stress reduction tips to help deal with anxiety-provoking experiences:

- **Put it in perspective**

Try to take a step back and ask: will this issue still matter in a year? In five years? If the answer is no, take a deep breath and try to move forward. Keeping things in perspective is crucial to managing stress.

- **Come up with a plan**

If there's a specific problem you need to fix, make a list of all possible solutions and pick the best one for your situation. Realizing that you have options and coming up with a concrete plan will have a direct effect on stress reduction.

- **Accept what you can't control**

Some circumstances are simply beyond our control, and we have to learn to accept them. Fortunately, we do have control over how we react to stressful situations. Staying calm and being willing to accept emotional support from others can help in managing stress.

- **Give yourself a break**

Have at least one relaxing activity every day. Listening to music, meditating, writing in a journal, or enjoying a soothing bubble bath. Taking time for yourself is important for both preventing and managing stress.

- **Get regular exercise**

Exercise is one of the best methods for managing stress because it can relieve both the physical and emotional effects of stress. Consider fitness choices that also deliver specific stress-reducing effects like yoga, tai chi, or Pilates.

- **Express feelings.**

If something's bothering you, don't keep it to yourself. Talk to people you trust, like friends, family, or co-workers, about what's on your mind. Even if you're not looking for specific advice, it usually feels good just to get feelings out into the open.

- **Set reasonable expectations**

Being busy is sometimes inevitable, but regularly taking on more than you can manage can cause unwanted and unwelcome stress.

- **Resolve issues before they become crises**

It's human nature to avoid unpleasant topics and circumstances, but if you're concerned about a brewing situation, whether it's at work or at home, address it early to keep it from becoming more serious, harder to solve, and more stressful. Problems are always easier to handle before they develop into full-blown calamities.

June 5

Coenzyme Q10 - Important Benefits
Chemo and CoQ10

In the very first days of my research I came across the importance of the CoEnzyme Q10 in relation not just to our cardiovascular system, but also to cancer. From the very beginning I am taking increased dose of CoQ10 which I believe has a big impact on the improvement of my blood. Here is more information on this very important enzyme.

CoQ10 is a naturally occurring compound found in every cell in the body where it plays a critical role in burning or oxidizing food for fuel. Our body levels of CoQ10 decline as we age leading to certain diseases and aging.

CoQ10 has a positive impact in battling cancer. If a patient chooses chemotherapy drugs, rather than less harmful alternative treatments, it appears the drugs are more effective battling cancer if CoQ10 is added as a supplement, even though irreversible damage is inflicted from the toxic drugs.

Japanese researchers at the National Cancer Center Research Institute in Tokyo wondered if CoQ10 could prevent cancers from beginning. They used a deadly carcinogenic chemical to induce colon cancer in rats. For one month the animals were fed an unsupplemented diet, while another was fed a diet containing CoQ10. The results were remarkable. At the first signs of colon cancer in the rats, they found the cancer was less than half that in the unsupplemented group.

The National Cancer Institute says laboratory and animal studies indicate that CoQ10 makes the body better able to resist certain infections and types of cancer and that CoQ10 may stop cancer cells from growing.

Integrative medicine advocate, Andrew Weil, advises to take 300 - 400 mg of CoQ10 daily as a possible hedge for survival in breast cancer patients, basing his recommendation on two reports from the 1990s by a Coenzyme Q10 manufacturer in Denmark. If you need to take large amounts try the ubiquinol form. Because CoQ10 is fat soluble, take it with small amount of fat.

There are also reports that CoQ10 supplementation increases survival of patients with cancers of the pancreas, lung, colon, rectum and prostate. CoQ10 has proven itself as a tissue-protecting antioxidant molecule enhancing brain and heart health. Now it seems this multi-faceted enzyme's role may have expanded to be a key nutrient in the battle to kill cancer cells and protect healthy cells from undergoing malignant damage.

CoEnzyme Q10 can supply oxygen from biologically active molecules. It is an internal part of the basic energy of the cell. Supplementing CoQ10 assists in the body's cellular respiration and energy production; it's that fundamental and that important! **Our bodies could not survive without CoQ10**, if body levels start dropping, so does our general health; scientists have estimated that once body levels of CoEnzyme Q10 drop below the 25% deficiency levels, many health problems begin to flourish, including cardiovascular problems, immune system depression, periodontal problems, lack of energy, and weight gain and it may be contributing factor to the aging process.

CoEnzyme Q10 is a nutrient necessary to the functioning of every cell in our bodies.

The quality of CoEnzyme Q10 is very important. The highest in quality is produced in Japan, there is no better. Before you purchase CoQ10, make sure it is a Japanese pharmaceutical grade, review the Certificate of Analysis and compare with others.

June 9

Top Superfoods – Healthy Skin

Healthy skin is a good sign of a healthy, cancer free, body. Below are 5 best superfoods and health supplements for creating youthful-looking skin and endorsing healthy life.

#1: Astaxanthin
Astaxanthin is carotenoid, a fat-soluble antioxidant. It protects the skin from sunburn, eliminating the need to use toxic sunscreen lotions, protects the brain from Alzheimer's disease, the eyes from UV light damage and the entire nervous system from oxidative damage. The best way to take astaxanthin is with a dietary source of healthy fats, like Omega-3 Oils.

#2: Ocean-Derived Omega-3 Oils
The best way to take astaxanthin is with high-quality omega-3 oils. Ocean-derived omega-3 oils are legendary for their ability to support the body's healthy response to inflammation, far more affordable alternative to dangerous prescription anti-inflammatory drugs. Before you purchase omega-3 make sure you read March 7th writing where I describe how to choose your vitamins and minerals. Marine omega-3 oils not only support healthy skin, they also support and enhance the health of the nervous system, cardiovascular system, respiratory system and many other functions of the human body, including moods and balanced brain function.

#3: Raw foods and fresh juice
Live foods support living, vibrant skin. Dead foods (processed and cooked) cause skin to age rapidly, and eating fried foods or animal products may cause your skin to break out with acne, eczema or various rashes. Consuming raw vegetable juice on a daily basis is a powerful way to support healthy skin. You'll notice the different in 30 days or less!

#4:Shellfish, Pumpkin Seeds and Zinc

Zink is an essential nutrient for skin repair and injury repair. When we are deficient in zinc our skin does not look as good as it could. Shellfish and pumpkin seeds are good natural sources of zinc.

#5: Clean Water

Adequate hydration is essential for optimum skin health. Far too many consumers are chronically dehydrated, and as a result they suffer systemic dehydration of their skin, which makes it look older, more wrinkled and less smooth. Don't buy bottled water as it creates a mountain of waste (plastic bottles). Furthermore, the Bisphenol-A in the plastic bottles has been proven so toxic that it was recently banned from baby bottles in Canada.

In summary, nutrition and hydration are the keys to healthy skin. Consume omega-3 supplements on a regular basis, take astaxanthin, drink plenty of clean water, and drink fresh juice on a regular basis. Also be sure to take in plenty of trace minerals through sources like Himalayan sea salt. Healthy salt allows your skin and body to hold on to water, lubricating joints, boosting nervous system function and smoothing out the skin.

I found another list of superfoods, created by Dr. Ariel Policano, that concentrate mostly on women's health. As a leading naturopathic physician with a special focus on women's health, Dr. Policano has over 15 years of experience using raw foods and superfoods to treat a wide variety of conditions. Having worked with health afflictions ranging from fatigue to breast cancer, she has crafted a definitive list of foods to emphasize in your diet for hormonal health, vibrant skin and healthy heart and bones:

- **Flax Seed**
  Excellent raw materials for the creation of health reproductive hormones.
  Anti-inflammatory.
  Good for healthy colon.
  Lignans improve hormonal balance.
  High "electron" food -- gives you energy and optimal cellular health.

Possible anti-cancer properties written about by Johanna Budwig.

- **Sprouts**
  Very nutrient dense.
  High protein.
  Good source of trace minerals.
  Broccoli sprouts have anti-cancer properties.
  Alkalinizing -- improves metabolism.
  Satisfies nutritional needs -- reduces appetite.

- **Kombucha**
  Supports excellent digestive health.
  Improves healthy gut bacteria that helps with production of serotonin, good mood hormone.
  Rich in enzymes -- helps energize the entire body, all organs, hormones and neurotransmitters.
  Rich in vitamin B-Complex.
  Alkalinizing -- improves metabolism.
  Has been used by some women as a part of a breast cancer treatment plan.

- **Goji Berries**
  Very high in antioxidants.
  High in Vitamin C.
  Complete protein containing all essential amino acids.
  Contains factors for human growth hormone.
  Rich in polysaccharide sugars for healthy immune system.

- **Coconut**
  Anti-bacterial.
  Anti-fungal.
  Anti-viral.
  Healthy source of saturated fats.
  Rich in electrolytes.
  Alkalinizing -- improves metabolism.
  Increases energy.

- **Marine Phytoplankton**
  Rich in chlorophyll.
  Alkalinizing -- improves metabolism.
  Cleansing.

Vegan source of EPA and DHA.
Many different carotenoids means strong antioxidant support.
Virtually all trace minerals in marine phytoplankton.
Great for balancing blood sugar.
Good for weight loss -- satisfies nutritionally, not as hungry.
Energy improvement.

- **Hemp Seed**
  Complete protein.
  Omega 3 and Omega 6 present in healthy ratio.
  Anti-inflammatory.
  Raw materials for healthy hormones!
  Contains chlorophyll for nourishment and cleansing.

- **Sea Vegetables**
  Thyroid health.
  Breast health.
  Weight loss.
  Cancer protection.
  High mineral content - good for blood sugar, focus and creativity.

June 13

Principles of exercise
Exercise cuts cancer risk 40%

One of the primary reasons exercise works to lower our cancer risk is because it drives our insulin levels down. Controlling insulin levels is one of the most powerful ways to reduce our cancer risks. It's also been suggested that programmed cell death is triggered by exercise, causing cancer cells to die.

It is becoming increasingly clear that a well-rounded exercise program is an important part of staying healthy. "Well rounded" means a program that includes the four primary types of exercise. Each type of exercise has very different and very specific impacts on our body.

1. Aerobic
2. Interval
3. Strength
4. Core

Aerobic: Jogging, using an elliptical machine, and walking fast are all examples of aerobic exercise. As we get our heart pumping, the amount of oxygen in our blood improves, and endorphins, which act as natural painkillers, increase. Meanwhile, aerobic exercise activates our immune system, helps our heart pump blood more efficiently, and increases our stamina over time.

Interval (Anaerobic) Training: Research is showing that the BEST way to condition our heart and burn fat is NOT to jog or walk steadily for an hour. Instead, it's to alternate short bursts of high-intensity exercise with gentle recovery periods. This type of exercise, known as interval training or burst type training, can dramatically improve our cardiovascular fitness and fat-burning capabilities.

Strength Training: As we age our muscle mass diminishes, and strength training is one of the best ways to replace the lean muscle mass that we've lost. Strength training also offers these additional benefits:

• Increases our bone density while lowering your risk of osteoporosis
• Lose weight (the more muscle you have, the more efficiently your body burns calories)
• Protects our joints from injury
• Helps maintain flexibility and balance
• Improves our stamina and lessens fatigue

Core Exercises: Your body has 29 core muscles located mostly in your back, abdomen and pelvis. Exercise programs like Pilates and yoga are great for strengthening your core muscles.

More than half of U.S. adults don't get the recommended amount of exercise, and one out of four don't exercise at all. When we begin to view exercise as a necessary component to our health, rather than a luxury, it becomes easier to find time for it during even the busiest days. Exercise will keep our energy level high, strengthen our immunity, improve our mood, and reduce the effects of negative stress, to name just a few benefits.

There are important points to remember for an exercise program to be effective. Make exercise habitual, progressive, and systematic.

- **Habitual:** Exercise at the same time of the day for at least 21 days, the time that it takes to either make or break habit.

- **Progressive:** Start with a few minutes a day; easily and steadily increase to 20-30 minutes of exercise each day.

- **Systematic:** Include a system of exercise that does three things:
  - Works the lungs with running, walking, swimming, and other aerobic exercises.
  - Stretches to muscles. It is better to stretch them after warming up.
  - Includes resistance work, such as a workout in the garden with digging and moving things and push-ups.

Bottom line:
Many people think of exercise as a tool for weight loss, but it is so much more than that. It is one of the most powerful tools available to drop your insulin levels, and elevated insulin levels are one of the primary drivers for high blood pressure, high cholesterol, diabetes, weight gain and many other chronic conditions. Properly performed exercise is far more powerful for controlling these symptoms than any drug yet developed.

Exercise can also:
- Reduce inflammatory chemicals in the body that promote the survival of precancerous cells
- Slow the aging process in your body
- Boost your immune system

June 16

Secret of a Joy-Filled Life

I just finished the book written by Tommy Newberry called "The 4:8 Principle". His idea is something I instinctively knew but needed to read and write about as another element of my transformation. Here is what caught most of my attention.

Approximately 90% of the thoughts we have today are repeats from yesterday and the day before. This is the primary reason why effecting permanent, positive life improvement tends to be met with such stiff resistance in most people. The secret of living an exceptional life tomorrow is purely a matter of thinking strong, joyful thoughts today. We are writing our own life story as a human being with each thought we think. **Thinking, talking, and worrying about what we don't want can never bring us what we want.** We never invite a thief into our house; so why would we allow thoughts that steal our joy to make themselves at home in our mind?

Positive circumstances do not come from negative thoughts. The most effective technique for the habit of positive thinking is developing a habit of asking, re-asking and answering positive questions, for example:

- What are the five things I am thankful for right now?
- What are five of my strengths or positive traits?
- What are five of my best achievements so far?
- Who are the five people who love me the most?
- What five things am I looking forward to in the next seven days?

To get these questions working for us, we place a copy where we can see them often, such as on a bathroom mirror, a night table, computer screen, fridge, or steering wheel in the car. We can not completely control the thoughts that are triggered from our surroundings, but we can unquestionably control what we choose to dwell on. When we change our focus, our circumstances change soon after – presuming of course, that we retain our new way of thinking. With each seed of thought, self-concept shifts toward our highest potential or away from it.

Any permanent progress in life starts on the inside and spreads to the outside. **All lasting growth begins with changes to the mental images we hold inside our head.** They ultimately spread to the outside and create permanent changes in our circumstances. Our self-concept is our distinctive combination of convictions, assumptions, life experiences, memories, feelings, and dreams for the future that are all bundled together to create the image that we hold of ourselves. If we become consciously aware of our self-concept, we can refine it to our advantage and tap into more of our potential. If, like most people, we're not aware of it, it is likely to work to our disadvantage and diminish our capacity for growth, contribution, and joy. What we do externally reflects what we are really like and what we are thinking internally.

Building Emotional Strength

We need to put the thought of perfection out of our mind, and emphasize daily improvement instead. It is important to build our emotional strength so that we can overcome the negative feelings that deplete our energy and minimize our potential for joy. Emotional strength refers to three things:

- emotional resiliency (speedy recovery from problems)
- emotional control
- emotional toughness

The foundation of emotional strength is mental well-being. When we focus our thoughts on what is noble and right, we develop our mental muscle.

Our task is to become proficient at interpreting the events of our life in such a way that we remain empowered to improve them.

The Laws of Emotional Strength

The Law of Attention

Whatever we dwell upon becomes increasingly prominent in our mind. For example, the more we emphasize our good health with both our silent thoughts and public speech, the healthier we feel. We will always feel what we dwell on. If our emotional life today is not where we ultimately want it to be, then our top priority should be shifting our attention to our blessings, to our strengths, and to the aspects of our life that are working. The flip side of the Law of Attention is that whatever we stop thinking about or turn our attention away from tends to drop out of our life.

The Law of Exchange
This simply means that we can do away with a negative thought only when we replace it with positive thought. We need to release the need to hang on to thoughts that haven't worked well in our life.

The Law of Reversibility
When we live purposefully, think rightly, serve generously, and forgive quickly, we are laying the groundwork for emotional victory. It is very important to start noticing our emotions and how they spiral quickly upward or downward. This peaked awareness shifts us from being the passenger in our emotional life to being the driver. To live life of maximum joy, we must learn how to minimize negative emotions so they will not dominate our life. When we change our focus, we change our life!

Our personal firewall
From inside the womb right up to the present moment, our character has been and will continue to be molded by our surroundings. If we neglect to take strategic control of those exposures, we'll find it's like building on the sand. We should realize that everything we read, watch, or listen to and especially the people we choose to associate with either bring us closer to joy or nudge us further away. What we let in our heart shapes what we believe, expect, and do.

For every outcome in our life, there is a thought or group of thoughts that are responsible. What we spread in thoughts, either useful or useless, manifests itself sooner or later in our circumstances. It is simply impossible to produce a result that has not first been formed in thought. "Guarding our heart" means protecting our subconscious from limiting, joy-suppressing beliefs. Our responsibility is to convince our subconscious that the joyful conditions we desire already exist. When we put garbage into our body, we pay the unpleasant short and long term consequences. When we allow garbage in our mind, we clog our potential for joy, satisfaction, and lasting success as well. We are the gatekeeper of our mind. To experience a life full of joy, we must reject the negatives and protect the positive.

Those who experience more joy don't necessarily have more to be joyful about; they think differently.

Habits that guard our joy:

Habit 1: Feed positive mental nutrition
This refers to deliberate inputs that come from what we read, watch, and listen to on a consistent basis. We should read books that raise interesting questions and inspire us to live and give in exceptional ways. When we are reading and listening to great ideas, then by default, we can't be filling our mind with mediocre inputs. We attract into our life the people, ideas, and circumstances that correspond with our habitual thinking. And three years from now, our family life, health, relationships, and finances will reflect what we have been feeding ourselves. We become what we think about most.

Habit 2: Start the day with joy
Focus on joy the first fifteen minutes after you wake up. If our morning doesn't start with joy, we will find it difficult to make a comeback later in the day. To start our day with joy, first we make a decision to do so, then we ask the positive questions mentioned before. Minutes invested in praying for wisdom will save days spent in overcoming mistakes.

Habit 3: Seal the day with joy
The absolute worst time to be negative, to be discouraged, to argue, or to deal with junk is right before bedtime. Just before the bedtime it is good to imagine our goals already accomplished, read an inspirational book, share a special moment with our loved one, or review our victories from the day.

June 17

Strategies for protecting mind

Here are more of the important points I took from Tommy Newberry's book.

Strategy 1: Focus on the right relationships
In life, it's far easier to be pulled down than lifted up. We should stay far away from people who shrink our dreams and who encourage the enemy called "good enough". Instead, we need to be around people who challenge us to constantly stretch, raise our standards, and pursue our biggest dreams. Negative people poison our outlook, exhaust our energy, and chip away at our potential for joy. Life is far too short to be captive by the negativity of others. We need to become alert to who is lifting us up and who is pulling us down.

Strategy 2: Memorize
Our conscious mind can hold only one thought at a time, positive or negative. The only way to eliminate a negative or counter-productive thought is to replace it with a positive, empowering thought. This is where memorization comes in. By committing scripture verses to memory, we begin the process of crowding out negative, limiting thoughts and replacing them with the tremendous power. A good start is to write down one verse each week on a three-by-five card and carrying it with us for the entire week, rereading several times a day.

Strategy 3: Visualize blessings
Imagine things as they could be rather than just as they are. We have been given power to have what we visualize, but we tend to visualize only that which we already have. And as long as we fix our mind only on what we currently have, we will very likely receive nothing more. Unquestionably, a clear vision for the future is a key prerequisite for reaching our full potential. Unfortunately many people spend their time visualizing what they don't want than what they do want. To get started, set aside four or five minutes every day to visualize yourself, in as much detail as possible, living a joy-filled life. We should see ourselves fully alive, loving our work, and having a strong, positive impact. Envision ourselves completely engaged and energized at home with our family. The two best times to

practice visualization are right before we go to sleep and just after waking in the morning. Take six or seven slow, deep breaths while imagining that our mind is completely free of old opinions, preconceived notions, our own knowledge, or entrenched negativity of any kind. Then fill our empty mind with perfect wisdom.

Strategy 4: Quarantine negativity
Negativity spreads like the flu – not just from person to person, but also from one area of life to the next. The powerful method of limiting the damage that negative situation and people can cause in our life is to 'schedule our negativity'.
Schedule a specific time each week to sit down and worry. When a worry comes to mind during the week, capture it in writing and remind yourself that you have set aside Tuesday at 7:00 pm do deal with it. That should be enough to get it of your mind temporarily so that you can return to and enjoy other activities. Make a note of how many real worries still remain Tuesday evening. Second, in your marriage or family life, you can schedule a weekly or daily 'issue time'.

Strategy 5: Establish ground rules
Become more intentional with your inputs – the things you allow into your heart.

1. Environmental. You are heavily influenced by your physical surroundings.
2. Association. You will gradually become like people you habitually spend time with.
3. Excluded alternative. When you say yes to the wrong inputs.
4. Non-neutrality. All inputs contribute to who you become as person! Nothing is neutral.
5. Attraction. Over time you will draw into your life the conditions, events, people, and possibilities that correspond with your thinking.

June 18

Gratitude

Gratitude is like a mental gearshift that takes us from turbulence to peacefulness, from stagnation to creativity. Gratitude brings us back to the present moment, to all that is working well in our life right now.

Gratitude is also an effective antidote to most negative emotions. The more we appreciate today, the more things we will notice tomorrow to be grateful for. On the flip side, the less appreciative we are today, the fewer blessings we will tend to acknowledge tomorrow.

Worrying or negative forecasting are obstacles to gratitude. Worry is the result of dwelling on what we hope doesn't happen but fear will happen! If we were predicting positive outcomes, we would not be worrying, right? The worst part of worry is that it displaces and then dissolves genuine thoughts of gratitude. We cannot worry and be grateful at the same time. When we focus on our blessings, our life feels abundant. When we focus on what's missing, life feels incomplete.

June 20

Thermographic breast screening

Thermography uses no mechanical pressure or ionizing radiation, and can detect signs of breast cancer years earlier than either mammography or a physical exam. It is the safest method allowing for breast cancer detection. Cancer cells are different than healthy cells. For one, they use a lot more sugar. For another, they give off a lot more heat.

The thermographic breast screening is simple, it measures the radiation of infrared heat from our body and translates this information into anatomical images. Our normal blood circulation is under the control of our autonomic nervous system, which governs our body functions. The technology converts infrared radiation emitted from the skin surface into electrical impulses that are visualized in color. The spectrum of colors indicates an increase or decrease in the amount of infrared radiation being emitted from the body surface. Mammography cannot detect a tumor until after it has been growing for years and reaches a certain size. Thermography is able to detect the possibility of breast cancer much earlier, because it can image the early stages of angiogenesis (the formation of a direct supply of blood to cancer cells, which is a necessary step before they can grow into tumors of size).

Current methods used to detect suspicious signs of breast cancer depend primarily on the combination of both physical examination and mammography. While this approach has become the main method of early breast cancer detection, mortality from this disease has gone relatively unchanged for 40 years. Since the absolute prevention of breast cancer has not become a reality as of yet, efforts must be directed at detecting breast cancer at its earliest stage. As such, the addition of Digital Infrared Imaging (Breast Thermography) to the frontline of early breast cancer detection brings a great deal of good news for women.

The bad news is that mammography causes the very disease it claims to "detect". Any supposed benefits of early tumor detection using mammograms is offset by the potential risk of radiation, including cancer.

June 22

Amino Acids

Often I hear and read about how important the amino acids are. I needed to find out more about this important part of our diet.

Amino acids are the building blocks of the proteins that are found in our bodies. Our body is mainly composed of proteins developed from amino acids. From twenty amino acids, the body manufactures more than fifty thousand types of protein. Amino acids are absolutely crucial for our good health.

Amino acids are broken down to two groups: essential and non-essential. Essential are those which cannot be made by our body, so we must get them from our diet. Non-essential amino acids are manufactured by our body. All of the amino acids perform vital functions in the body, it is important to get a variety of protein in our diet. The proteins in foods that contain all of the essential amino acids are called complete proteins. The complete sources of protein are in dairy products, meat, fish, poultry, eggs and soy.

There is a common misunderstanding that it's very difficult for vegetarians and vegans to eat the right combination of amino acids. Although there should be a little planning involved, we can still easily get all of the essential amino acids without eating meat or dairy. It's not necessary to combine all the amino acids at every meal as long as we are eating a good variety of protein-rich foods on a daily basis. To eat a good combination of amino acids without animal products, we should include plenty of these foods in diet:

- Raw Nuts (almonds, walnuts, Brazil nuts)
- Raw Seeds (pumpkin, sunflower, sesame)
- Beans (lima, chickpeas, pinto, navy)
- Whole soy foods (tempeh, edamame)
- Whole grains (buckwheat, quinoa)
- Vegetables (red potatoes , onions, mushrooms, broccoli)

When it comes to getting the right amino acids, the work isn't hard but the payoff is still enormous: a healthy body and mind that can function at their best.

June 29

Radiation update

Last week I finished the set of 25 radiation sessions that were concentrating on the entire right breast. Today I had the first out of eleven sessions concentrating on the area where the tumor was. In the beginning of the last week my doctor, with help of radiation technicians, decided on the exact spot that will receive the radiation. While they were choosing the area, I have mentioned that my scar is away from where the tumor was, that the tumor was higher because Dr. Jane did not want my scar to be exposed, therefore she made her cut low and went up under my skin to remove the tumor. My comments were not taken seriously, when I came home I realized that marks on my breast were not including the area where the tumor was, only the scar was included. Next day I had my weekly visit wit Dr. Catherine; one more time I brought to her attention that the cavity left after tumor's removal is not in the marked circle. She apologized and next day changed the parameters of the localized radiation. I am not sure if every patient pays as much attention as I do to what is being done to their body.

The eleven radiations are my final sessions. Once the radiation is over I will be pronounced cancer free, and will enter the remission. Dr. Catherine said that for patients with breast cancer there are no tests available (blood, urine or other) that can prove that the cancer is gone. The diagnosis that I am cancer free will be based on the fact that I have followed the conventional cancer protocol by agreeing to surgeries and the radiation. Unfortunately this is not good enough for me. I need more than just certificate of completion of radiation to believe that I am cancer free. This week I will send my urine to Philippines for testing, as I did the two times before. I am hoping for a response with number less than 50.

My whole right breast and approximately an inch outside looks like I have the strongest suntan ever. Sometimes I feel a little fatigued, I am loosing hair and it seems to be much drier. Otherwise I feel great. My appreciation for life is greater than ever, each day more peace flows to my mind, and I don't take anything for granted.

June 30

Personal Foundation

Because our self-concept is our personal foundation, every effort to make it stronger will pay multiple rewards. Here are steps to build the strong personal basis:

Recognize the true source.
Too many people base their self-worth on what others think about them. But, if we depend on others for our self-worth, is it even accurate to call is self-worth? Beware of idolizing other people's opinion. Needing approval from others is an immobilizing trap. It is saying that someone else's opinion of us is more important. It may be helpful in certain situations to remind ourselves quietly, "What you think of me is none of my business".

Focus on strengths.
Emphasize originality by highlighting special gifts and talents. Surrender the idea that we need something or someone else to make us complete. Focus on unyielding self-development. Ask repeatedly, "How am I better, stronger, and wiser today than I was yesterday?"

Eliminate negative self-talk.
Changing the way we communicate with ourselves changes our self-concept faster than any other single method. Speak only what we seek, as we are already living the life of our dreams. Start programming the mind by first disciplining our mouth. Cut out, one by one, every expression or remark that is inconsistent with the person we want to be.

Practice extreme self-care.
When we neglect the wise habits of good health, we make ourselves much more vulnerable to the worst aspects of human nature. When we become drained, run down, or fatigued, we tend to get stuck in the negative.

Dwell on the person we want to become.
Visualize best self. Develop a meticulously clear personal mission statement that lays out the full potential in this lifetime. Enlarge the mental territory. Use imagination, not memory, to achieve this faith-driven perspective. Meditate frequently on the character qualities we want to see.

Act with joy now.
Anyone can be happy when circumstances are wonderful, but joy is different. Joy is proactive happiness. It is the learned capacity to display faith ahead of time by means of the daily

mental attitude. Proceed, moment by moment, with gratitude as if all our prayers have been answered.

July 1

About Vitamin E

The disease fighting powers of vitamin E are enormous. Not only can it enhance cardiovascular health and immunity, but it can also improve skin health, fight cancer, protect from Alzheimer's, and keeps us strong. Taking vitamin E might save over 200,000 women annually from dying of heart disease, says Dr. Maret Traber, worldwide authority on vitamin E.

You may have seen headlines implying vitamin E has no significant health benefits and could be harmful, but this is not true, as says Dr. Andreas Papas and many others. These studies involved people taking one type of synthetic vitamin E, which is quite different from the full spectrum of natural vitamin E. The current research not only confirms vitamin E's efficacy, but new studies are also uncovering more specialized applications for the unique forms of vitamin E. Since it is practically impossible to get protective amounts of vitamin E from food, taking supplemental vitamin E is essential to achieving vibrant health and longevity. But know that all vitamin E supplements are NOT created equal. Many contain synthetic vitamin E, and many do not contain all of the various types of natural vitamin E that the body requires. Make certain that your supplement contains both natural tocopherols and tocotrienols in their natural forms if you want to get the most out of what E has to offer. It is recommended to take between 400-800 IU on regular basis. Because of my situation, I take 1,000 IU a day.

You can tell what you're buying by carefully reading the label. Natural vitamin E is always listed as the "d-" form (d-alpha-tocopherol, d-beta-tocopherol, etc.). Synthetic vitamin E is listed as "dl-" forms.

July 5

Hidden Dangerous Ingredients in Groceries

Many food additives have been studied and linked to various diseases. Becoming informed about the additives in everyday food items can make for an easier shopping experience and healthier food choices for everyone.

The top three most dangerous ingredients found in groceries are listed below. Read labels, look for these, avoid them!

1) **Sodium nitrite** -- causes cancer, found in processed meats like hot dogs, bacon, sausage. Used to make meats appear red (a color fixer chemical).

2) **Hydrogenated oils** -- causes heart disease, nutritional deficiencies, general deterioration of cellular health, and much more. Found in cookies, crackers, margarine and many "manufactured" foods. Used to make oils stay in the food, extending shelf life. Sometimes also called "plastic fat."

3) **Excitotoxins** -- aspartame, monosodium glutamate (MSG) and others. These neurotoxic chemical additives directly harm nerve cells, over-exciting them to the point of cell death, according to Dr. Russell Blaylock. They're found in diet soda, canned soup, salad dressing, breakfast sausage and even many manufactured vegetarian foods. They're used to add flavor to over-processed, boring foods that have had the life cooked out of them.

When foods are processed not only are valuable nutrients lost and fibers removed, but the texture, natural variation and flavors are lost also. After processing, what's actually left behind is a bland, uninteresting "pseudo-food".

At this point, food manufacturers must add back in the nutrients, flavor, color and texture to processed foods in order to make them tasty, and this is why they become loaded with food additives.

Many Food Additives Increase Your Risk of Cancer:

- BHA and BHT
  It is often used in making baby and water bottles. The chemical then leaches into the liquids inside. BPA is also used in the lining of tin cans, and is being found in canned foods. Even if you are eating otherwise healthy green beans or peas - if it is canned, it is likely contaminated with BPA. BPA is dangerous even in small amounts.
- Propyl Gallate
- Trans Fats
- Aspartame.
- Acesulfame-K
- Food Colorings (Blue 1, 2, Red 3, Green 3, Yellow 6)
- Potassium Bromate

These additives are in countless products from baked goods and chewing gum to chicken soup base, cereal, luncheon meats, vegetable oils and potato chips. If you eat a highly processed food diet, you are therefore potentially exposing yourself to cancer-causing toxins at every meal!

Avoid products made with any of the crops that are Genetically Modified Organizm GMO. Most GMO ingredients are products made from the "Big Four": corn, soybeans, canola, and cottonseed. These are commonly found in processed foods. Some of the most common GMO Big Four ingredients in processed foods are:

Corn - corn flour, meal, oil, starch, gluten, and syrup. Sweeteners such as fructose, dextrose, and glucose. Modified food starch.

Soy - soy flour, lecithin, protein isolate, and isoflavone. Vegetable oil and vegetable protein (these may come from other sources but it`s better to safe than sorry).

Canola - canola oil (also called rapeseed oil).

Cotton - cottonseed oil.

Sugar - avoid anything not listed as 100% cane sugar.

Recently, Jeffery Smith, the well known exposer of GMOs, has produced a "NON-GMO SHOPPING GUIDE". This shopping guide is free to download. Go to www.centerforfoodsafety.org and/or www.healthiereating.org to download it. Below is Jeffery's basic guideline.

Four Ways to Avoid GM Foods
1. Buy organic
2. Only buy products that carry a Non-GMO label
3. Only buy products listed in the non-GMO shopping guide
4. Avoid products that contain these at-risk ingredients: soy, corn, cotton,canola

DID YOU KNOW THAT:
- Feeding children hot dogs increases their risk of brain cancer by 300%.
- Food companies now "hide" MSG in safe-sounding ingredients like yeast extract or torula yeast.
- Many Florida oranges are actually dipped in an artificial orange dye in order to make them more visually appealing It's the same dye that's been banned for use in foods because of cancer risk.
- Girl Scout cookies are still made with hydrogenated oils that contain trans fatty acids.
- Many so-called "healthy" or vegetarian foods also contain the very same offending ingredients as conventional groceries.
- Eating just one serving of processed meats each day increases your risk of pancreatic cancer by 67%.
- Any artificial color additive causes behavioral disorders in children. And that 80% of children diagnosed with ADHD can be outright cured of the condition in two weeks by avoiding certain ingredients.
- The #1 ingredient in Slim Fast meal replacement shake (powder form) is sugar.
- Some guacamole dips don't even contain avocado. Instead, they're made with hydrogenated soybean oil and artificial colors.

July 7

Detox – Simple Ways

The relationship between unhealthy eating and the development of disease is undeniable. When most people get a cancer diagnosis their doctors are quick to prescribe drugs and harsh treatments such as radiation, chemotherapy, and surgery. All of these treatments have a traumatic effect on the body opening it up to a whole host of other problems. Holistic health practitioners, on the other hand, will often recommend detoxification methods such as cleansing to eliminate cancer from the body.

The message is: Try everything you can naturally before so that you never regret. Medical procedures such as surgery, radiation, and chemotherapy consider be the last resort.

Detox, short for detoxification, is the purification of the body by removing toxins. Our bodies naturally eliminate toxins through the skin, liver, kidney and lungs. However due to the massive amount of toxins in the air, water and food supply today our bodies are unable to "keep up" with the amount of toxins invading us daily. This leads to fatigue, weight gain and health problems. Therefore it is necessary for us to detoxify our bodies in order to reclaim the health and vitality.

Why do 95% of diets fail?
The diet industry is a multi-billion dollar industry. These companies are in the business to make money, not to make us thin and happy. They spend more money on advertising and marketing than they do on actually developing products that work. Think about it: if the products worked, the diet industry would be out of business!

The only way to lose weight and get healthy is to know why we are fat in the first place and then take the necessary steps to make a change.

Why are we fat?
Toxins! From the food we eat to the air we breathe to the water we bathe in, toxins invade our body daily. Toxins are stored in our body fat. Toxins cause our livers to become sluggish and to

not function properly. This causes our organs to stop metabolizing fat effectively and we gain weight. The more toxins we accumulate, the more weight we gain. Even worse, the more we weight, the more toxins we store.

How do we lose weight and reclaim our health and vitality? Detox Tips:

1. Eat organic fruits and vegetables
Conventional fruits and vegetables are full of chemicals that harm our body. Organic food is grown without the use of pesticides and artificial fertilizers. The sooner we stop polluting our body, the sooner we will start to look and feel healthier.

2. Eat kosher meat
When we eat a burger the growth hormones that were given to the cow are passed on making us grow and gain weight! Organic meat is produced without giving the animal antibiotics or growth hormones. Buy certified organic meat and only eat free-range chicken. Your body will thank you.

3. Do a juice fast
The juice fast essentially means we drink juice throughout the day, every day. The juice must be fresh and organic. This can be done for 3 days, 10 days or 30 days. It depends on the level of discipline, and health goals. If you have never done a juice fast before then you will start seeing results right away!

4. Add apple cider vinegar to your diet
It can be used in salad dressing or drank with water. Apple Cider Vinegar helps detoxify the liver. Take 2 teaspoons of apple cider vinegar mixed in water before every meal to aid in weight-loss or add it to hot water with raw honey to drink as a tea. A hot bath prepared with a cup of apple cider vinegar and a cup of Epsom salts withdraw toxins out trought the skin.

5. Drink green tea
EGCG, an antioxidant contained in green tea, helps the body burn fat. Antioxidants such as vitamins A, C, E, and the polyphenols found in green tea also help the body reduce the time that toxins stay in the system.

6. Dry-brush before you shower
Dry brush the skin before every shower. This removes dead skin cells and toxins helping lose weight and have glowing skin.

7. Get a shower filter
The tap water can contain pesticides, toxic bacteria, viruses and traces of human and animal waste. Every time we take a shower or drink out of the tap we are ingesting dangerous toxic chemicals. Filtering water also improves your hair and skin!

8. Add fiber to your diet
Fiber keeps the meal moving along the gastrointestinal tract and helps flush the body of metabolic waste. Fiber also keeps the energy levels high, and slows the rate of carbohydrate digestion, which helps maintain the blood sugar levels.

9. Use only natural and organic beauty products
Most of the beauty products are full of toxins, preservatives, and even poisons. These are put in our beauty products in order to give them a longer shelf life and thus give the company more profits. Using organic products guarantees that we will not be putting toxins into the body every day.

The more toxins we eliminate from the body, the more weight will be lost and the more healthy we'll become!

Master Cleanse
Another way to detox is using the master cleanse. Use fresh squeezed lemon juice, Real Maple Syrup, water and cayenne. Make two quarts. One quart would be the juice of about 4 lemons (6-8 oz), maple syrup start with 2 oz if not sweet enough add more, water to make one quart, taste for sweetness and lemon-it should taste like good lemonade only less sweet, then add as much cayenne powder as you can take (work up the amount). By the glass it would be approximately the juice of one lemon, a few teaspoons or more of maple syrup, water and a dash of cayenne. You can find more information on line about this by googling: master cleanse and/or Stanley Burroughs who developed this back in the 1920's or 1930's. It is quite cleansing and will make you feel energized. Make sure to use real maple syrup not Aunt Jemima's and the like which is just high fructose corn syrup and artificial flavoring. You might

read that people go on the Master Cleanse for 2-4 weeks; I prefer 3-5 days, or even just mornings till noon or 1:00 PM.

July 8

About Liver

Don't mess with liver. It serves a vital function in almost every system in our body; from hormone and digestive enzyme production to blood filtration and the last stop in chemical digestion of medications. Along with the heart, brain and pancreas is an organ that we cannot live without.

Our liver is a hardworking three to five pound organ that sits under our right rib cage. Unlike most organs with just a handful of jobs in your body, our liver has over a thousand jobs, and daily detoxification is one of its most important ones. Our liver is the prime detoxification organ responsible for the hundreds of man-made chemicals that most of us put in and on our bodies each and every week. Chemicals and genetic alterations are new to the food supply, and that it takes the body many thousands of years to biologically adapt to anything new. With all of these chemicals entering our body many times each day, the liver, our prime detoxification organ, is often the hardest hit.

When our liver is overwhelmed with incoming chemicals, two things happen. First, those chemicals and toxins back up in our body and become trapped inside because the liver didn't have the resources to deal with them. When there is an accumulation of these chemicals and toxins in the body, health problems are often the result. Second, weight loss becomes difficult because in addition to being our prime detoxification organ, the liver is our prime fat burning organ.

The solution is simply to cleanse our body and liver, to remove the stored toxins from the liver and to reduce body's toxic load in general. In today's chemical driven world, internal body cleansing should be as commonly regarded as washing hands.

Coffee enema is a very effective way to cleanse and care for the liver. Coffee enemas work to cleanse the liver and body because the caffeine in the coffee dilates or opens our bile ducts, which is the pathway from the liver to the colon. When the pathway from the liver to the colon is open, the liver has an open path to dump its stored toxins into the colon for removal with the enema, which it happily does.

July 9

Coffee Enema

I decided to introduce one more way of detoxification to my process of healing; the coffee enema. Enemas and colonics have been used for hundreds of years and are regarded as safe. Coffee cleansing enemas have a chemical makeup that is stimulative. The enzymes in coffee help the liver carry away toxins; the liver and the colon receive significant cleansing. The detoxification process is fast and the backlog of yet to be detoxified substances is minimized. Bring 3 quarts (3 liters) of filtered water to boil, add 2 flat tablespoons of organic coffee per quart, continue to boil for 5 minutes, then turn the stove off, leaving the pot on the hot burner allowing to cool to a comfortable temperature. Poor half this solution into an enema bag, follow regular enema directions, repeat. I will do one enema every 10 days; however, I will not forgo licensed medical attention as the alternative. I am already in contact with two trained colon hydrotherapist, Clear Path Therapies and Lake Travis Wellness Center. Prescription by a medical doctor is required. Each of the two places can provide the prescription for a fee.

July 10

What are Free Radicals?

Free radicals are toxins, from the environment or by-products of digestion or drugs, believed to cause or worsen many diseases. They steal electrons from our cells, creating weak unhealthy cells in the process. When our cells are weak, we eventually become weak and/or sick. The way to keep free radicals from damaging our cells is to zap them with antioxidants. Antioxidants, present in many foods, are molecules that prevent free radicals from harming healthy tissue.

The problem starts when these free radicals attack our healthy cells and cause them to weaken and become more susceptible to health disorders. Plus, this can also have a profound effect on how we age. But as part of normal functioning, our body is capable of keeping free radicals in check and naturally neutralizing them, unless we:

- Eat a diet consisting mostly of processed junk food, including unhealthy oils, artificial sweetener, MSG
- Cut corners on getting enough sleep on a daily basis
- Ignore our need for regular exercise
- Find ourselves under a great deal of stress
- Expose ourselves to a high number of environmental free radicals, such as industrial pollutants, household chemicals, cigarette smoke

Exposing our body to these types of conditions may overwhelm it with free radicals and cause damage.

So what can we do?
First we must address the unhealthy habits listed above.

The next step is to find ways to fortify our healthy diet with antioxidant rich food that contain natural antioxidant compounds called polyphenols. Polyphenols existing in fruits and vegetables contribute to the antioxidant capacity of our diet much more even than vitamins. Unfortunately, conventional growing methods that use pesticides block the production of flavonoids.

We don't want to miss out on polyphenol flavonoids because they can:

- Improve our memory and concentration
- Boost the effectiveness of vitamin C in our antioxidant network
- Regulate nitric oxide – a potent free radical that regulates our blood flow

141

- Help promote our healthy heart
- Bolster our immune system

To take advantage of the highest potency flavonoids and rich antioxidants, choose organically grown fruits and vegetables; refer to February 26 for list of fruits and vegetables that do not have to be organic. Fresh organic foods are important not only for what they give us, higher levels of antioxidants and nutrients, but also for what they don't give us... exposure to pesticides, herbicides, and non-organic fertilizers. Besides, they taste 100% better!

Food sources of antioxidants:
- All berries, but watch out for too much sugar. Moderation is the key when eating fruit.
- Broccoli, cabbage, kale, mustard greens, beans, artichokes, and onions, to name few.
- Oregano and other herbs ranked even higher than fruits and vegetables. Find fresh, organic source; for example fresh garlic is 1.5 times stronger than dry garlic powder.
- A potent polyphenol found in grape skins and seeds called resveratrol.

Resveratrol
Studies show that resveratrol may increase the lifespan in human cells. So, it could be a determining factor in extending your longevity. Resveratrol helps reduce oxidative stress damage to our cardiovascular system by neutralizing free radicals. And it helps support our body's natural defense system.

Plus, resveratrol benefits you by how it...

- Protects our cells from free radical damage
- Helps us keep your blood pressure within the normal range
- Keeps our heart healthy and helps improve blood vessel elasticity
- Boosts our protection against the spread of abnormal cell activity
- Helps us better control the aging process

July 11

Reasons for eating Raw Foods

In 2006 a raw food diet study was made conducting 500-participant survey of raw food eaters. The study showed that people who ate 80-90 percent raw foods showed significant improvements in immunity, digestion, allergies, weight, disease, energy, and mental and emotional well-being.

#1 - Energy
Eating raw foods increases our energy. There are a few reasons for this; one is that our body does not have to spend as much energy digesting our food. Raw foods contain enzymes, and these enzymes help your body break down food.

#2 - Cleansing
Elimination improved dramatically on a raw food diet. People who reported having two or more bowel movements per day increased from 25 percent to 78 percent. Having a properly functioning digestive tract is vital to maintaining optimal health.

#3 - More Time
Preparing raw foods takes a lot less time, compared to cooked foods.

#4 – Weight Lost

#5 - Environment
Producing meat costs an incredible amount of energy and food. This food could be used to feed starving nations and let nature recuperate. A meat-based diet also requires 7 times more land than a plant-based diet.

#6 - Mental Health
One of the most dramatic and encouraging areas of improvement occurred in mental, emotional and spiritual health.

Caution About Teeth
When you start eating raw foods, you have to pay special attention to your teeth. Make sure you rinse your mouth after every fruit meal, especially smoothies. There are many natural mouthwashes on the market today that are excellent.

How to eat to get the full benefit out of this important part of our lives? Here are a few exercises:

- Say grace. Offering thanks for the delicious food and abundance you enjoy calms you and focuses your mind on the meal ahead.
- Consider the food. Take a moment to enjoy the smell and look of the food before grabbing your fork.
- Eat slowly. Savor each bite, chewing slowly, so you can experience the food's subtle flavors.
- Pay attention. Even when eating on the go, you'll feel more satisfied if you concentrate on your food instead of trying to work, read, or watch TV while eating.

July 15

End of Radiation

I waited for this day long time, total of 36 radiation sessions. The last two weeks were not so good. I had started to react by diarrhea and fatigue. I was told that this will continue for at least two more weeks. Yet, considering the three surgeries and radiation, I am amazed with my body's condition, the healthy way I feel, and my understanding and positive reaction to the circumstances attached to the last six months of my life.

My last visit in Oncology was touching. Jill and Jennifer, the radiation technicians, hand made for me a beautiful card telling me how much they will miss my positive energy and how courageous I am; they sprinkled bouquet of confetti all over my head. Then I met with Dr. Catherine (radiation oncologist) who gave me 'Certificate of Radiation Completion' and told me that I am in remission now. I was also told to make an appointment with Dr. Beth (chemo oncologist) for Tamoxifen and Dr. Jane (surgeon) for mammogram. I have decided to avoid both appointments and continue my natural ways of healing. I am afraid of Tamoxifen and mammogram and will not go against my instincts.

I am not done yet, I will not consider myself in remission until I have an evidence that cancer left me. Physically I feel it is gone, but my mind needs a proof. My urine sample is ready to be sent. It will go to Philippines tomorrow, once I receive results I'll know where I truly am.

July 18

Beliefs about Health and Illness

Dr. James Chestnut, who was honored in 2007 as "Chiropractic Educator of the Year" by the International Chiropractors Association, applies a different approach to his practice, combining genetics, nutrition and exercise with the science of personal change and empowerment, he offers a fresh perspective on what "health" really is.

The current conventional model, which views "health" as freedom from disease symptoms, is a fundamental flaw of current medicine. If people believe that health is related to genetic predetermination, there is no logic or hope for wellness or prevention. In addition, the conventional medicine presents as prevention – early detection. Pap smear or a mammogram is called "prevention," which of course is absurd, because they can not prevent anything. If our model is that everything flows from the gene down and we can't do anything about this, then really, there's no such thing as wellness or prevention.

The state of health is mainly determined by how we eat, move, and think; not what our genes show.

We are responsible for our own health.

Without this fundamental change of consciousness, alternative therapies are not being considered; instead people believe that disease will happen, and when it does, it will be treated by drugs. The truth is that to actually create health, we must get right down to the root cause.

Dr. Chestnut says that the natural therapies are useful but they are only used by the people who are sick. The goal should not be to treat or have therapy for a particular illness at all. The whole goal should be to restore health. And that's a very different pattern.

As soon as we truly understand that our genes do not predetermine our health and longevity, it becomes self-evident that it's our lifestyle choices that trigger disease and sets the bar for our level of health.

It's imperative to realize that it's NORMAL to be healthy! Our lifestyle choices should be aimed at living up to our potential; to optimize our health, rather than trying to run from inevitable disease.

People believe that disease is not normal and that drugs can cure it. This cultural belief system was created and paid for by the pharmaceutical industry to the tune of tens of billions of dollars a year. Our lifestyle choices will either help or delay the healing process. Supplying drugs never was, and never will be, the solution. This disease-based pattern is what's being taught in medical schools. It's the popular belief system of the last century.

So by waiting until we get sick and then deciding to battle our illness with conventional medicine is the same old pattern. Make a difference now, turn to natural therapies; eat whole foods, exercise, and think positive!

Below is more about the conventional vs. naturopathic doctors described by Dr. Pizzorno.

In health care there are two basic philosophies: one is kind of the interventionist philosophy seen by conventional doctors, where the role of the doctor is to diagnose that disease and treat that disease. And the other side is more of the natural oriented kind of practitioner who believes their primary role is to promote the health of the patient rather than specifically treat disease.

Naturopathic doctors treat diseases from the perspective of helping the body get healthier so that the body can get rid of the disease. For example, a medical doctor might use a drug, an antibiotic, to kill an infection. Naturopathic looks at why is that person's immune system not working the way it's supposed to, and look at what diet, herbal, lifestyle changes they need so that immune system will work properly, and not only will that current infection go away, but there is less chance of infection in the future.

It is important to recognize that conventional medicine has strengths. If somebody has an accident, or obvious bacteria infection such as TB and pneumonia, conventional medicine has some great tools. But for the day to day practice of health care, conventional medicine tools are weak, and the more we change our focus from disease diagnosis and treatment focus to understanding why people are sick and how to help them to become healthy, we start realizing that the drugs aren't very useful. The great strength of natural medicine is our ability to understand why people are sick and deal with the underlying cause of their illness. More and more conventional medical doctors are getting frustrated with drugs, because by far, the majority only relieve symptoms, they don't deal with the underlining cause why that person is sick.

The longer we use the drug the longer the disease progresses, the more difficult it is for the body to re-establish normal health.

Most of side effects from commonly prescribed drugs are due to nutritional abnormalities included by the drug. And this is one reason why using them with natural supplements can be so effective, because if we know what nutritional abnormalities are being inducted by the drug, by providing extra amounts of those nutrients, we can help mitigate a lot of side effects of the drug.

Fact: Between 80% and 85% of cancer today is inducted by dietary abnormalities both deficiencies and excesses, and environmental toxins people are exposed to. The numbers come form medical literature.

To find a naturopathic doctor go to www.naturopathic.org,

July 20

Cancer Poem

This poem was written by a terminally ill young girl in a New York Hospital.

SLOW DANCE
Have you ever watched kids on a merry-go-round?
Or listened to the rain slapping on the ground?
Ever followed a butterfly's erratic flight?
Or gazed at the sun into the fading night?

You better slow down.
Don't dance so fast.
Time is short.
The music won't last.

Do you run through each day on the fly?
When you ask how are you?
Do you hear the reply?
When the day is done do you lie in your bed
With the next hundred chores running through your head?

You'd better slow down
Don't dance so fast.
Time is short.
The music won't last.

Ever told your child, we'll do it tomorrow?
And in your haste, not see his sorrow?
Ever lost touch, let a good friendship die?
Cause you never had time to call and say, 'Hi'
You'd better slow down.
Don't dance so fast.
Time is short.
The music won't last.

When you run so fast to get somewhere
You miss half the fun of getting there.
When you worry and hurry through your day,
It is like an unopened gift.... thrown away.
Life is not a race.

Do take it slower
Hear the music
Before the song is over.

July 22

Trans Fats

Trans fat is the worst kind of fat for our health because it both raises bad cholesterol and lowers good cholesterol. Trans fat is formed when oil is hydrogenated, or processed to become solid.

When hydrogenated fats like margarine and shortening were first invented, they became the ingredient of choice because they were cheaper, more shelf-stable, and thought to be healthier than butter. It was only recently confirmed that this fat is especially unhealthy.

Trans, or hydrogenated fat, is found in stick margarine, vegetable shortening, and fried foods. Until recently, it was also found in most commercially packaged baked goods, crackers, pastries, cookies, and many other products. However, in 2006, when it became mandatory for companies to list trans fat on food labels, many manufacturers changed their formulas to reduce the amount of trans fat their products contain. You can now find soft margarines that boast "trans fat–free" on their label, and many packaged baked goods are advertised as trans fat–free. However, some foods may contain small amounts of trans fat even if they list zero grams of trans fat in the Nutrition Facts panel. To avoid trans fats completely, check the ingredients list on a product for "hydrogenated" or "partially hydrogenated" oil of any type. If such an ingredient is present, there is still some trans fat in the food. And if the trans fat ingredients are near the top of the list, drop the box and run the other way!

If there are no truly trans fat–free foods in your regular grocery store, check out a health food or whole-foods store. And be on your guard in restaurants — unless the menu specifies otherwise, many fried foods are still prepared with hydrogenated oils.

Remember:

1. When a fat gets cooked for as little as 3 minutes at relatively low temperature, it not only kills the inherent enzyme in that food but it also flips the hydrogen bonds into a trans fat.
2. The molecules of cooked fat solidify like a piece of gum then get stuck on the inside of the artery walls, which can trigger a heart attack.

The end result of the hydrogenation process is a completely unnatural fat that causes dysfunction and chaos in our body on a cellular level and have been linked to:

- Cancer: They interfere with enzymes your body uses to fight cancer.
- Diabetes: They interfere with the insulin receptors in your cell membranes.
- Decreased immune function: They reduce your immune response.
- Problems with reproduction: They interfere with enzymes needed to produce sex hormones.
- Obesity
- Heart disease: Trans fats can cause major clogging of your arteries.

July 23

Oils – From Most Unsaturated to Most Saturated

Before commenting on specific oils I need to better understand what saturated and unsaturated fats are.

	Saturated Fats	Unsaturated Fats
Derived from:	Mostly from animal products	Plants
Health:	Excessive consumption is not good because of their association with atherosclerosis and heart diseases.	Unsaturated fats are considered good to eat if you are watching your cholesterol
Commonly found in:	Butter, breast milk, meat	Avocado, soybean oil, canola oil, olive oil
Recommended consumption:	Not more than 10% of total calories per day.	Not more than 30% of total calories per day
Form:	Solid at room temperature	Liquid at room temperature
Cholesterol:	Saturated fats increase LDL (bad cholesterol)	Unsaturated fats increase HDL (good cholesterol)

Unsaturated fats have been divided into two groups. Monounsaturated fats such as olive oil, and polyunsaturated fats such as sunflower oil.

It's important to choose the right saturated fats, like real raw butter and extra virgin coconut oil. Avoid highly processed fats and especially hydrogenated oils, which have been proven to cause heart disease, cancer and a slew of other conditions.

One of the reasons we need good saturated fat is because our brain consists mainly of fat and cholesterol, and it needs saturated fat more than any other kind. Even the brain-friendly omega-3 fatty acids can't be utilized without saturated fat.

Healthy Fats

- Extra-virgin olive oil: provides more monounsaturated fat than any other oil, it is considered the healthiest. Buy only extra virgin oil and cold pressed. Not recommended for cooking.
- Flaxseed oil: A rich source of healing oil, flaxseed has been cultivated for more than 7000 years. Essential fatty acids work throughout the body to protect cell membranes, keeping them efficient at admitting healthy substances while barring damaging ones. Flaxseed oil is an excellent source of omega-3s: Just 1 teaspoon contains about 2.5 grams, equivalent to more than twice the amount most people get through their diets.
- Extra-virgin organic coconut oil, good for cooking

Unhealthy Fats

- Omega-6 oils (corn, safflower, sunflower, peanut, canola, and soybeans)
- Margarine: avoid, one molecule away from plastic.
- Chicken fat, lard, beef fat: too saturated. Avoid them entirely or minimize consumption. Unlike vegetable fats, they contain cholesterol.
- Butterfat: the most saturated of all the animal fats and contains the most cholesterol. Minimize consumption of butter, ice cream, and whole milk products. Use butter made only from raw milk.

July 30

Urine Test Results (Third)

Today is my birthday and today I finally received response from Philippines. My urine sample was sent exactly two weeks ago, I was waiting on the results impatiently. The news is good, I am almost cancer free! The natural ways I have added to the conventional protocol are helping me immensely. In only one month the number indicating the strength of cancer dropped significantly and now is very close to 50. Once I am below 50 I am cancer free.

Dear Alexandra,

Your latest HCG test result on 7-30-09 is:

Index + 4, **(51.4 Int. Units)**

This is within the positive range. It shows a decrease as compared to the last result on 5-11-09**(53.0 IU).**

Wishing you the best of health, I remain
Sincerely yours,
EFNavarro,MD

In summary; the first result came back February 25th and was 52.2. The second sample came back May 11th, just after my three surgeries, and it was 53; this proofs that conventional ways of treating cancer pushed me behind. Today's result is 51.4. To get down below 50 I will continue everything I am doing plus go on the Miracle Mineral (MMS) protocol, which helped many people. I will write about this healing method in following days.

August 2

Diet Guidelines

The following dietary habits may contribute to health problems:
- A diet that is predominantly acid-forming.
- A diet that is too high in animal fats and proteins.
- A diet that contains many harmful additives.
- A diet that is too processed and refined.

In addition, these lifestyle factors may affect well-being:
- Too much stress.
- Too little exercise.
- Too little or too much sunshine.
- Too little fresh air.

Unhealthy dietary and living habits contribute to many health problems, including:
- Fatigue and insomnia
- Excess weight and cellulite

- Malnutrition
- Cravings and bingeing
- Dark circles under the eyes
- Headaches
- Depression
- Mental problems
- Behavioral problems
- Reproductive disorders
- Pre-menstrual tension
- Premature aging
- A host of more serious diseases such as: autoimmune diseases, diabetes, heart disease, cancer, and more.

The diet industry in the U.S. is worth $35 billion. Large food companies provide most of the mainstream dietary information to the public. Dietetics at most universities is funded by these corporations and pharmaceutical companies. In schools, children are taught the food pyramid and how eating all things in moderation will keep them in proper health.

People are focusing on energy (calories) over nutritional value. So they remove the fat and add more artificial additives and flavors, ignorant of the impact this may have on their health. When overweight people focus on becoming healthy, the weight drops off naturally without having to weigh and measure themselves or their food.

Guidelines
1. Remember the K.I.S.S. Principle: "Keep it straight and simple."
- Eat food that the human body is biologically designed to eat.
- Health is freely available to everyone.
- Use basic common sense and make better choices.
- The body will repair and heal itself if it is fed the right, natural foods.

2. Check Out the Research
For example, for years, the dairy industry has been telling people that milk, milk products, yogurt, and cheese will prevent osteoporosis (brittle bone disease), yet the countries that consume the most milk and milk products have the most osteoporosis cases. The countries that consume the least dairy

have the least brittle bone disease. Look at independent research based on real people.

3. Learn to Listen to Your Body
In learning to listen to our body, we can tune into our natural body cycles. When we are asleep, the body automatically steps up their repair and cleansing operation. To assist the body in this it needs to be fed properly.

When we eat a very heavy evening meal that is also poorly combined, the body is using most of its energy to sort out the contents in the stomach rather than repairing, cleansing, and rebuilding. They we wake up after eight hours of sleep feeling totally exhausted.

The Five Perfect Health Steps

STEP 1: Eat One Fruit Meal a Day
Raw fruit eaten on its own, on an empty stomach, digests in less time than other foods and leaves an alkaline residue in the bloodstream. Some fruit might be acidic before it enters the body, and might digest in a more acidic environment than other fruits, but it is never acid-forming in the body or bloodstream unless it is eaten in a wrong combination with other foods.

Fruit is easily digested because the nutrients are readily available for absorption and assimilation directly by the body.
- The sugar in fruit is a simple sugar, or monosaccharide.
- The protein in the fruit is in its broken-down form (amino acids).
- Vitamins and minerals (includes calcium and iron in every single fruit) are in the most usable form.
- The fats are in the form of fatty acids.
- It cannot be broken down any further.

STEP 2: Snack on Raw Fruit or Vegetables Before Eating Refined Sugar or Heated Fats.
Fruit is very high in vitamins and antioxidants and is a valuable source of carbohydrates and vegetables are a plentiful source of many minerals and antioxidants. Vegetables are also alkaline in the bloodstream. Most independent research states that

155

people need to be following a 75 to 80 percent alkaline-forming diet.

Research from Britain shows that the higher the alkaline environment in the brain, the higher the IQ. And the way to create a higher alkaline environment in the body is to eat more alkaline-forming foods.

See March 3 for table of alkaline foods.

For sufficient fats, the body needs one of the following six sources of fat, plus a flax blend and barley grass juice daily:
- avocado
- 1/4-1/2 cup of raw unsalted nuts or seeds
- 5-10 olives in brine
- 1-3 tablespoons of cold-pressed falxseed oil.
- Dark green leafy vegetables, whole or juiced, or 2-3 teaspoons of dried barley grass juice

STEP 3: Start All Cooked Meals with Raw Vegetables
Start all cooked meals (especially lunch and supper) with a medium plate of raw, uncooked vegetables. For ideas, visit: www.mary-anns.com. British nutritionist and immunologist Jennifer Meek found that starting cooked meals with raw vegetables prevented destruction of white blood cells, which is important in maintaining a healthy immune system.

STEP 4: Food-Combining (See March 16 Table)

STEP 5: Try to Eat Animal Protein No More Than Three Times a Week
Vegetarians should try and include at least a quarter to half a cup of raw, unsalted nuts every day. Legumes are difficult to digest as they are generally cooked. Cooked protein is more difficult to digest. Soaking legumes overnight in filtered water before cooking makes them more digestible. Keep red meat down to a maximum of one time per week.

August 3

Food Pyramid

Below is the Food Pyramid from Ray Strand's book "Healthy for Life". This pyramid is science based and is primarily focused on the consumption of good carbohydrates, good proteins, and good fats. Although this is good guide for majority, I have eliminated from my diet the two top sections and red meat, except for an occasional Bison meat, organic red potatoes and organic cheese made out of raw milk.

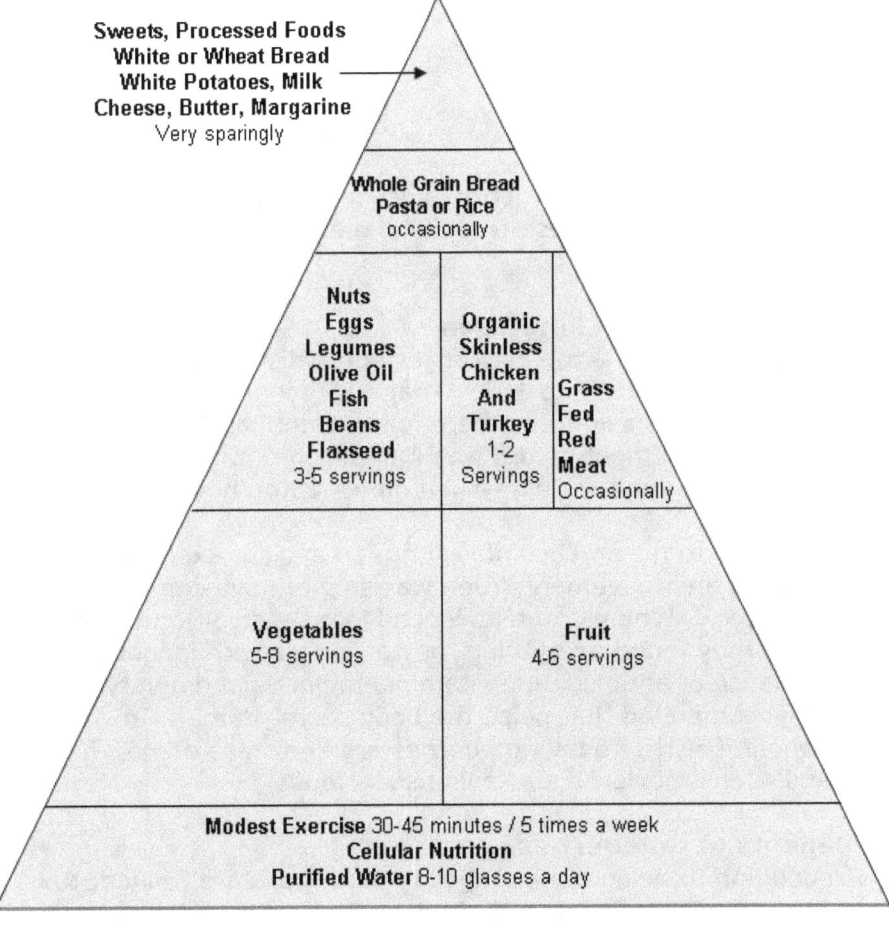

Remember, carbohydrates are not the problem, processed and high-glycemic carbohydrates are our main enemy. However, eliminating or significantly decreasing all carbs from our diet will create even greater problems. Good carbohydrates are the main source of our vitamins, antioxidants, and minerals as well as the fuel source the body prefers (glucose).

The proper balance of three major macronutrients is 40-50% of calories from carbohydrates, 30% calories come from fat, and 20-30% calories come from protein.

August 8

About Goji Berries

What is a Goji Berry?
The goji berry is the fruit of the Lycium barbarum plant, and has been used in Chinese traditional medicine for thousands of years.

The Legend of Li Ching Yuen
Li Ching Yuen was a master Chinese herbalist who was said to have lived from 1677 to 1933. That's 256 years! The story of his long life was said to be mere folklore until an Imperial Chinese government record was found from 1827, congratulating one Li Ching-Yuen on his 150th birthday.

In addition to his practice of Qigong, an ancient exercise of breathing and movement, Yuen was said to have consumed goji berries daily. When scientists looked into the health properties of goji, they found everything they associate with longevity; an abundance of antioxidants, vitamins, minerals and a very special compound that helps the body secret Human Growth Hormone (HGH). Today goji berries are known as one of the world's most powerful anti-aging superfoods.

Benefits of Goji Berries
In addition to being a top longevity food, gojis are thought to be the most nutritionally rich fruit on Earth. Gojis contain more iron than spinach, more beta carotene than carrots, and more protein than whole wheat. Gojis are packed with 18 amino acids,

eight of which are the essential amino acids, including isoleucine and tryptophan. Plus goji berries are one of the highest antioxidant containing fruits in the world, typically containing 2-4 times the amount found in blueberries.

Goji berries are also an excellent source of minerals, such as zinc, iron, copper, calcium and phosphorous, as well as vitamins B1, B2, B6 and E. Gojis contain key nutrients that promote healthy vision, and have been recommended for thousands of years in Chinese medicine to improve eyesight.

One of the most fascinating aspects of goji berries is their ability to help the body produce Human Growth Hormone (HGH). The production of HGH is considered by many to be our body's own internal Fountain of Youth, and decreasing levels of HGH have been linked to accelerated aging. For example, a seventy-year-old produces only one-tenth of the amount of HGH as a twenty-year-old.

August 21

Why We Should Eat Raw Honey

Long before what we refer to as civilization was born, honey was a food prized above all others in many traditional cultures. Ancient peoples in Spain, India, Egypt and all over the world knew that honey supplied a unique richness of nutrients. But far from squeezing honey out of cute little plastic containers, these people were eating their honey freshly harvested from local bee hives, untouched and untainted by civilized man. They worshiped pure, raw honey, and for good reason.

Why Raw Honey:
- Raw honey contains bee pollen, which many leading nutritional experts refer to as a potent superfood. Among bee pollen's many benefits are allergy relief, detoxification, anti-cancer properties, increased energy, amino acids, vitamins and thousands of beneficial enzymes.

- Raw honey is one of the richest natural sources of amylase, an enzyme which facilitates the proper digestion of carbohydrates. This makes raw honey an excellent companion for toast or oatmeal. This essential enzyme is lost the moment honey is heated, since amylase converts to starch when exposed to heat.

- Propolis, a material bees use for constructing their hives, is another beneficial part of raw honey. Propolis is believed to have antioxidant, antimicrobial and even anti-cancer properties. It is said to boost the immune system and improve the health of the liver as well.

Tips for Enjoying Raw Honey:
- Remember, processed honey has been extensively heated and filtered to make sure it's the same clear, golden liquid we've all come to expect. This is essentially honey stripped of all its goodness, and contains none of the beneficial nutrients listed above. Raw honey will be opaque and creamy with a slightly crystallized texture. It's ideal for spreading on bread or scooping up with a spoon.

- Pay close attention to labeling to make sure you are getting a quality raw honey. It should be completely unprocessed and unheated. The valuable enzymes in honey are preserved only if the honey is never heated above 105 degrees, although purists claim that for honey to be truly raw, it should never be heated at all.

- On the same note, raw honey should only be added to foods after they have been cooked and never before, since any exposure to heat risks destroying the beneficial nutrients in the honey.

- Raw honey stored in sealed, airtight jars will not spoil. It is a very stable food that becomes finer with age, just like a quality wine. Open jars will stay fresh for at least several months. Even then, raw honey will simply ferment, not spoil. Fermentation enhances the benefits of raw honey, although some do not prefer the taste.

- While all sugar is not created equal - and in fact many would say raw honey is superior to all other forms of sugar - in the end, raw honey is still, well, sugar. Eaten in excess, it can still have a negative impact on blood sugar levels and can cause related health problems. However, in moderation raw honey is a wonderful health food that is as nutritious as it is utterly intoxicating.

Lesson learned: when buying honey make sure you look for Raw Honey, NOT other.

September 7

Colon and Health

After years of research and experience with patients, Dr. Group shared the best secret for good health: a clean intestinal tract. Most disease-causing toxins enter the body through the intestines and then spread into the bloodstream. Some amount also enters through the skin and respiration. These toxins come from air, food, and water, and accumulate in the intestines, causing bowel problems as well as disease.

People should be having three to four bowel movements every day, with the time from eating to eliminating being from 12 to 18 hours. Te reality is that in Western countries like the United States many people only have a few bowel movements per week and the transit time of the food averages 38 hours. This problem affects up to 20% of the population and explains the occurrence of laxatives, which actually damage bowels.

A toxic colon causes many problems in the body. For one, it cannot absorb as many vitamins, minerals, and other nutrients during digestion. Additionally, toxins will leak through holes in the intestinal walls (leaky gut syndrome) and spread to other parts of the body through the bloodstream.
Cleansing our bodies is one action we can take now to improve our health.

What does colon cleansing?
- Removes the built-up matter from the intestinal lining, thereby removing the reason for these conditions
- Increases the frequency of bowel movements
- Makes stool easier to pass
- Keeps toxins from moving into the bloodstream

- Speeds up the time eating and eliminating, removing toxins more quickly from the body

Explanation of the body's basic natural cycles:
- Elimination: 4am to noon; good time to eat fresh raw fruits
- Energy: Noon to 8pm; good time for raw vegetables and starches
- Regeneration: 8pm to 4am; time for quality sleep and healing

Refer to July 7 for ways to detox and July 8 for coffee enema.

September 11

Reduce Toxins from Drugs and Stress

Most drugs prescribed by traditional doctors treat symptoms but don't cure the cause. Constipation will likely be a side effect of prescription drugs, which means that toxins are building up in the colon and cause additional health problem later on.

Antibiotics are one of the most over-prescribed and very dangerous medications. They kill off the beneficial bacteria in the colon as well as the bacteria they were meant to destroy. Which the 'good bacteria' no longer protecting the colon, the harmful bacteria can go wild and spread to other parts of the body. If you have taken antibiotics, be sure to take probiotic supplement to re-establish the beneficial bacteria.

Vaccines, amazingly enough, contain chicken embryos, preserving heavy metal, along with other toxic ingredients. These are especially damaging to young children whose bodies are small and still growing. Both colon and liver cleanses are necessary to get rid of the damage these drugs have done. Natural alternatives to these are available.

Stress can manifest in our lives as sleepless nights, headaches, poor concentration, intestinal ailments and dozens of other symptoms. These can be caused by stress hormones, poor diet, fast eating, and lack of exercise. Instead, try meditation, chiropractic adjustments, massage, improved diet and exercise, and time outdoors to create a healthier life. Go back to March 1, June 1, June 16, and June 17 for ways to control mind and stress.

How to reduce toxins from heavy metals and radiation

We are exposed to heavy metals such as mercury, aluminum, lead, and cadmium frequently through canned food, toxic fish, dental fillings, and deodorant. These can come into the body via the skin, the mouth, or the nose. They cause chemical reaction that releases free radicals which then impair cell function. Be sure to avoid aluminum in cookware, PVC plastics, and pesticides.

Everyone is aware of the dangers of nuclear radiation but few are aware of low-level radiation, also called electromagnetic field radiation (EMF). These come from power lines, cell phones, computers, fluorescent lights, clock radios, and even hair dryers. EMFs are known to mutate chromosomes and damage cells. A Swedish study noted that cell phone use increases the risk of brain tumor by 240%. The risk includes carrying it on your body as well as holding it against your head. People who work electrical wiring also are at risk.

Radiation can be minimized by
- Replacing fluorescent lights
- Using a speaker with cell phone
- Setting up a Safe Space Clearing Device
- Using as few electronic appliances as possible
- Turning off electrical equipment when not in use

How to reduce toxins from parasites

Parasites are not just of the microscopic variety, but can also be bacteria, fungi, viruses and long worms.
- Giardia – in contaminated water; causes diarrhea
- Tapeworms – in undercooked meat and fish
- Pinworms – from contaminated clothing, hands, bed sheets

- Hookworms – from walking bearfood on contaminated ground

To avoid these bugs:
- Wash fruits and vegetables
- Cook all meats and fish thoroughly
- Drink water from safe sources
- Wash hand frequently
- Keep you living and work areas clean
- Wear shoes outdoors
- Take a probiotic supplement regularly

September 17

Beets as an Alternative Cancer Treatment

Beets are one of nature's wonder foods. They've recently been found to increase stamina during exercise by 16% and that's just the tip of the iceberg. Beets are known to break up cancers and tumors, and they're known to do so faster than the body can eliminate them.

In fact, in the 1950's, Dr. Ferenczi of Csoma, Hungary used beets exclusively to break up tumors in the body. He had considerable success, and tumors were often completely eliminated. However, he found if patients stopped drinking quantities of beet juice, tumors often reappeared. Dr. Ferenczi recommended drinking about a quarter gallon (2.2 lbs) of beet juice daily to break up tumors, and results were often seen in a few weeks or months.

Because beets can break up tumors so rapidly, it's wise to combine this therapy with other detoxification methods, like colon and liver cleansing, to help your body dispose of the waste released when cancers are broken down.

The key cancer fighting ingredient in beets is called betacyanin; it's what gives red beets their bright purple reddish color. Beets have also been found to increase detoxifying compounds in the body and make it easier for the body to detoxify itself in general. This, of course, adds to health.

Knowing this, perhaps you'll want to start consuming beets regularly? Juiced beets are great, and you can add sliced raw beets to any salad. Cooked beets are also a fabulous side dish or main meal.

An estimated forty percent of the population is expected to have a problem with cancer, and tumors often grow for twenty years before they are diagnosed. Eating beets a couple of times a week, or more, can offer considerable protection from this serious problem.

Remember that only red beets will do the trick, and be sure they're organic. These days some beets are genetically altered, and genetically modified plants. Of course, nothing genetically altered will make you well; genetically modified foods will only make you sick.

Raw Beet Juice, use all organic:
1. Combine 1/3 cup beet juice, little ginger, clove of garlic, celery juice, and carrot juice.
2. Combine juice of 1 apple, 1 carrot, 1 beet, ½ lemon (optional)

September 19

Decrease Risk of Cancer - Vitamin D

There are 30,000 genes in our body and vitamin D has been shown to influence over 2,000 of them. That is one of the primary reasons it influences so many diseases, from cancer and autism to heart disease and rheumatoid arthritis.

The misguided advice to avoid the sun may very well be responsible for many cases of cancer each year. By getting more appropriate sun exposure, our body will naturally produce vitamin D, which has been found to be major key that can help prevent a vast number of major diseases. For example, studies have shown we can decrease the risk of cancer by more than half simply by optimizing vitamin D levels with sun exposure.

Vitamin D is a fat-soluble vitamin that is vital for optimal health and disease risk reduction. It's found in food like raw milk, eggs, fish and pure orange juice, but we only get an average of 250 to 300 international units (IU) of vitamin D per day from dietary factors alone, which is rarely enough to maintain optimal levels. Recent research has found that it takes 5,000 IU of vitamin D per day to have a significant impact however, about 10 percent or more of the people reading this needs significantly more. Some people require over 30,000 units of vitamin D a day to reach therapeutic levels of 25 hydroxy D in their blood. Fortunately, vitamin D is also made in our body after exposure to ultraviolet rays from the sun.

Another function of vitamin D in our body is to maintain normal blood levels of calcium and phosphorus. During the summer months, we get enough vitamin D from just spending some time outside every day. Our body can produce about 10,000 IU of vitamin D per day with full body exposure, about 5,000 IU with 50 percent of our body exposed, and as much as 1,000 IU with just 10 percent of our body exposed. Some also worry that if they are in the sun that they will overdose on vitamin D. However this is not the case, and here's why: when we're exposed to the sun, the UVB rays cause vitamin D to be produced in our skin while the UVA rays in the sunlight will tend to destroy excessive levels of vitamin D circulating in our body. It is somewhat of a natural failsafe mechanism that prevents overdosing.

It's always wise to have vitamin D level tested, especially prior to taking oral supplements of vitamin D. This is best done by a nutritionally oriented physician. It is very important that they order the correct test as there are two that closely resemble each other: 1,25(OH)D and 25(OH)D.

The best is to take vitamin D on empty stomach.

Top foods containing vitamin D:
- Shiitake & Button Mushrooms
- Mackerel
- Sockeye Salmon (wild)
- Herring
- Sardines
- Catfish

- Tuna
- Cod Liver Oil
- Organic Eggs

September 26

Lemon

Lemon is one of my favorite fruits; it has been known for its therapeutic properties for generations.

Over and over I read and hear that drinking pure water with lemon squeezed in it is one of the healthiest beverages. The primary benefits are the wonderful alkalizing properties of the lemon juice. By having lemon squeezed in the water I create a beverage that raises my body's pH.

Benefits of lemon:

1. Lemon being a citrus fruit, fights against infection.
2. Lemon is an antioxidant which deactivates the free radicals preventing many dangerous diseases like stroke, cardiovascular diseases and cancers.
3. Lemon lowers blood pressure and increases the levels of HDL (good cholesterol) .
4. Lemon is found to be anti-carcinogenic which lower the rates of colon, prostate, and breast cancer.
5. A few drops of lemon juice in hot water are believed to clear the digestive system and purify liver as well.
6. Lemon juice acts as a natural hair lightener and skin bleach which reduces the pigment melanin and prevents the risk of chemical allergic reactions which is common with hair dyes and bleaches.
7. Lemon juice is given to prevent the common cold.
8. Lemon juice is given to prevent or treat urinary tract infection and gonorrhea.
9. Lemon juice used for marinating seafood or meat kills bacteria and other organisms present in them, thereby prevents many gastro-intestinal tract infections.
10. A table spoon of thick lemon syrup everyday relieves asthma.

To increase the cleansing action of lemon water, add the following ingredients:
- a pinch of cayenne pepper
- a small amount of freshly grated ginger
- a ½ teaspoon of organic maple syrup (optional)

September 27

Top Foods for Healthy Immune Response

Here are some good points I found in an article written by Dr. Mercola. He summarizes what I have included in many days of this book. I believe that repetition irons the information we want to keep as par of our behavior. This is why I return to this book often, to remind my self of the importance of many lessons that I have learned over long time.

So, avoiding processed foods, grains and sugar will go a long way toward strengthening our immune system. Selecting foods that are loaded with specific immune boosting nutrients helps even more. Below are foods that help protect, this list is certainly not exhaustive.

Unpasteurized Grass-Fed Organic Milk
Raw organic milk from grass-fed cows contains beneficial bacteria that prime our immune system and can reduce allergies. It is an outstanding source of vitamins, especially vitamin A, zinc, and enzymes. Raw organic milk is not associated with any of the health problems of pasteurized milk such as rheumatoid arthritis, skin rashes, diarrhea and cramps. Raw milk also contains beneficial fats that will help our immune system.

Although raw milk availability is limited in the US depending on where you live, you can locate the source closest to you at RealMilk.com.

Fermented Foods
If we are serious about boosting our immunity, then adding traditionally fermented foods is essential;

however, watch out for highly acidic foods such as pickles or sauerkraut. One of the most healthful fermented foods is kefir. Kefir is an ancient cultured, enzyme-rich food full of friendly microorganisms that balance our "inner ecosystem" and strengthen immunity. Besides kefir, use yogurt (watch for sugar).

As we already know, friendly bacteria have a powerful, beneficial effect on our gut's immune system, our first line of defense against pathogens, and aid in the production of antibodies.

Raw Organic Eggs from Free-Range Chickens

Before you wrinkle up your nose, raw eggs are an inexpensive and amazing source of high-quality nutrients that many people are deficient in, especially high-quality protein and fat. A single egg contains: nine essential amino acids, six grams of highest quality protein, lutein an zeaxanthin (for our eyes), choline for the brain, and naturally occurring B12.

As long as you have a good source for fresh, organic raw eggs, you need not worry about salmonella. To find free-range pasture farms, try your local health food store, or go to http://www.eatwild.com or http://www.localharvest.org.

Locally Grown Organic Vegetables

When it comes to fighting off pathogens, we simply can't do any better than eating a variety of fresh, organic and raw vegetables for the vitamins, minerals, antioxidants and enzymes they contain. Veggies that we choose should be fresh. The nutrient value drops to practically zero once a fruit or vegetable is canned.

Blueberries and Raspberries

Blueberries and raspberries rate very high in antioxidant capacity compared to other fruits and vegetables. Wild blueberries in particular are potent immune boosters. They contain powerful phytochemicals, such as anthocyanin, which is the pigment that gives blueberries their color. And they are lower in sugar than many other fruits. They must be organic.

Mushrooms (more on mushrooms in May 6 writing)

Mushrooms strengthen our immune system because they are rich in protein, fiber, C, B vitamins, calcium and other minerals, and even vitamin D -- one of the only foods that can provide you with this essential immune strengthener. Mushrooms also contain powerful compounds called beta glucans, which have been long known for their immune enhancing properties. The beta glucans in medicinal mushrooms (especially Reishi, Shiitake and Maitake) are notable for their ability to activate our immune system and fight cancer.

Chlorella (pure green algae)

As foods go, chlorella is nearly perfect. Chlorella is a single-cell freshwater algae that acts as an efficient detoxification agent by binding to toxins, such as mercury, and carries them out of your system. It is the chlorophyll in chlorella that makes it so powerful. Chlorophyll helps us process more oxygen, cleanses our blood and promotes the growth and repair of our tissues.

Green Tea

The Chinese have known about the medicinal benefits of green tea since ancient times, using it to treat everything from headaches to depression. Journal of the National Cancer Institute published the results of an epidemiological study indicating that drinking green tea reduced the risk of cancer in Chinese men and women by nearly sixty percent. University of Purdue researchers recently concluded that a compound in green tea inhibits the growth of cancer cells. There is also research indicating that drinking green tea lowers total cholesterol levels, as well as improving the ratio of good (HDL) cholesterol to bad (LDL) cholesterol.

Matcha is the most nutrient-rich green tea and comes in the form of a stone-ground powder, completely unfermented. The best Matcha comes from Japan and has up to seventeen times the antioxidants of wild blueberries.

Herbs and Spices

There are simply too many good ones to summarize; here are few that deserve special mention.

Garlic: it's antibacterial, antiviral and anti-fungal. We should be eating garlic every day. One of the best things about garlic is that bacteria, viruses, and yeast build up no resistance to it, unlike with synthetic antibiotics.

For optimal benefits, garlic should be fresh since the active ingredient is destroyed within one hour of smashing the garlic cloves. In other words, garlic capsules are basically useless. Garlic has been shown to lower LDL, lower total cholesterol, lower blood pressure, reduce your risk of blood clots and stroke, and even prevent insect bites, including mosquitoes and ticks.

Turmeric: general immune system booster due to its high antioxidant capacity, and an anticancer agent as well; turmeric is 5 to 8 times stronger than vitamins C and E.

Black Pepper: increases the bioavailability of just about all other foods.

Oregano: a strong antioxidant; one tablespoon of oregano has the antioxidant capacity of one medium apple.

Cinnamon: found to kill E. coli and many other bacteria; also has anti-inflammatory compounds

Cloves: good anti-inflammatory.

Dr. Mercola had an interview with herbalist Donnie Yance, who shared his basic remedy for flu. Make this special tea from a combination of herbs that synergistically cause your body to sweat, which is very desirable if you want to eradicate a virus from your system. And then drink it hot and often:

Elderflower (this has been used for hundreds of years for flu)
Boneset
Yarrow
Linden
Peppermint
Ginger

Fact about eggs:
Eggs are one of the healthiest foods one can eat. Eggs actually lower the risk of heart disease, not raise it as health officials like to say. The numerous studies have supported the finding that eggs have virtually nothing to do with raising cholesterol. The International Journal of Cardiology showed that, in healthy adults, eating eggs every day had no negative impact on cholesterol levels or cardiac risk. Eggs are an incredible source of high quality nutrients, especially protein and unsaturated fat. One caveat: choose the highest quality free-range organic varieties. If possible, purchase your eggs from the farmer directly, or if you live in Austin, let me know. I have free ranged chickens that I feed organic veggies and I share their eggs for free. The best are raw eggs, which I cannot force myself to eat. Second best are boiled, avoid fried.

September 30

The Last Day

Today is approximately nine months since I was diagnosed with breast cancer. My life is very much different than it was before; it is better even though I was faced with the life threatening news. This news made me who I am today because I was strong enough to find positive aspects in my situation and act accordingly. The life changes I made based on the knowledge I passionately absorbed still amaze me: I had seven colon hydrotherapy sessions; removed a tooth with the root canal; went on a totally new diet with plenty of raw organic foods; I am on a new exercise routine; the set of friends I interact with on regular basis does not include negative characters; I clean my house, my dishes, and my clothes using 'green' products; I use natural self care products. Even my pets eat natural foods, and my cat Lola has a natural litter. Tomorrow I have the first appointment to remove the mercury filling that I have in three teeth. I am very proud of myself!

I pray that I'll be able to share my experiences with women that were diagnosed with cancer so they can have clear choices going forward. I also hope that I will inspire other woman to live a preventive lifestyle. The apathy and incompetence of the cancer establishment are no secret, yet millions of cancer patients each year have little choice. We are told by our oncologist that if we refuse conventional therapy, we will die. Some of us are cured, many are not. The "cured" that went through the entire conventional protocol often suffer lifelong damage and side effects that increase their risk of future disease. This is why understanding all choices is very crucial in making decisions.

Knowing we have many choices will eliminate the fear when we are told that we have cancer and there are a multitude of breast cancer causes that we have absolutely no control over. That pumping toxic chemicals into our body, radiation, or just cutting body pieces off is NOT the only way to restore our health. I have agreed to three breast surgeries and radiation before knowing what I know now; I will always believe that the natural ways of healing are the best and that we need to take responsibility for our own health before agreeing to the drastic methods that are introduced to us as our only hope for curing this disease. I would not come out of cancer as fast as I did if I was not diligent about natural ways in addition to the conventional methods doctors convinced me to undertake.

Overcoming cancer is a process of reversing the conditions that allowed the cancer to develop and going after the cancerous cells. Many natural ways of killing cancer that I have learned will never be too much, only too little. The more I am doing, the more ways I am attacking cancer, the greater are my odds for success. I will continue my natural treatments for another year to give my body the time and energy it needs to fully recover. After all, the natural ways do not have negative side affects. They only strengthen the body and give it a fighting chance to recover from cancer's overgrowth and invasion of our cells.

The principle of life transformation is that life change comes from the inside out. I believe in accepting 100% responsibility for everything that happens to me, this is why I am making incredible progress in my life.

Here are just few lessons I have learned during my journey:

- I am fully responsible for my own health, my daily habits create my great health.
- I envision perfect health and happiness every morning and before I go to sleep.
- Negative thoughts produce acid throughout the entire tissue system. Pure and happy thoughts build beauty and optimal health. I become what I think about the most.
- Holding on to past injuries serves no purpose in creating a successful future.
- I honor myself by saying NO to things I don't want to do.
- I avoid too many acidic, not alkaline rich foods, they have impact on the way I think, feel, and behave.
- I avoid excessively cooked and processed foods, they take away energy and feeling alive.
- No more sugar, except for an occasional glass of wino. I switched to only organic wino, with no sulfites added. All wines have natural sulfites; the sulfites artificially added are what is toxic and gives us a headache.
- Food is very potent medicine, as long as it is free of pesticides and hormones. I eat whole foods, eliminating refined sugar, refined flower, refined salt, and pasteurized milk.
- 80% of our immune system lives right in our digestive tract; I take probiotics, enzymes, and fiber every day.
- Only natural, not synthetic vitamins and minerals are worth taking.
- When I exercise I breathe deeply to bring as much oxygen to my body as possible.
- When I garden, I no longer hide from sun, I soak the vitamin D every chance I get.

174

- I have learned to tune in and listen to my body; I understand it and react to its signs.
- I moved my microwave to the laundry room. I stopped using it months ago and did not want to look at it any more. I don't even use it for pet's food. I keep my microwave only for zapping kitchen sponges to kill bacteria. Microwaves seriously deplete the nutrients in our food; destroy the structure of vitamins and enzymes, altering the structure of food which may cause pathological changes in our body.
- Finding the purpose and meaning in the occurrence of my cancer helped me find the way to cure it. Cancer is my body's reaction to what was done to it.
- Cancer is not a localized condition. My whole body is involved in healing cancer, the whole body needs to be healed, not just the place where the tumor was removed.
- Cancer will only kill me if I let it!

Well, this is it. I have reached the point where I feel like I have enough information to take care of my life. I will miss writing; however, I will always stay connected with the latest information related to my wellbeing, it is now part of me.

Good luck to you! Stay strong once you choose change, a new life path will unfold in front of you and you'll feel better than you ever thought you could, and remember, Love Wins!

Few Good Recipes

Healthy Banana Bread
Most banana bread recipes are saturated with butter and sugar.
This one uses a small amount of olive oil instead - which is
much better for the heart – and raw honey, which of course
means lots of flavor and no refined sugar. I make this bread
almost once a week and share with my friends and family.

3 very ripe bananas
1/2 cup raw honey
3 tbsp olive oil, plus a little more for oiling the loaf pan
1 tsp pure natural vanilla extract
1 1/2 cups gluten free flour
1 1/2 tsp natural baking soda
1/4 tsp Himalayan sea salt
3/4 cup chopped raw walnuts

Heat the oven to 350 degrees. Lightly oil a loaf pan.
Mash the bananas and mix with the honey, oil and vanilla
extract.
Stir together the gluten-less flour, baking soda and salt. Add
the nuts.
Blend the two mixtures and spoon into a lightly oiled loaf pan.
Bake for 45 minutes, or until center is set.

Banana Papaya Pudding
Smooth, creamy and filling, this pudding is also delicious with
two pitted prunes or figs blended in. I serve this as dessert.

1/2 ripe papaya (approximately 1 cup) peeled and seeded 1
banana peeled and cut in chunks

Put the papaya in a blender and blend just enough to break up
the fruit. Add the banana; blend until smooth. Eat immediately.
Serves 1.

Tangy Lime Dressing
This dressing tastes great on fresh green vegetable salads and
is truly alkaline.

1/4 cup fresh lime juice
1 1/2 tsp raw honey
1/2 tsp Himalayan sea Salt
1 tbsp chopped onion or minced chives
2 tsp finely grated ginger
1/4 cup extra virgin olive oil

Pour the lime juice into a small bowl and whisk in the honey and sea salt until dissolved. Add the chives or onions along with the ginger. Slowly add the Avocado oil in a steady stream, whisking until thoroughly mixed.

Red Pepper Vinaigrette
This is high in flavor salad dressing but low in calories (no oil) for those who watch their weight.

1/4 cup apple juice from organic apples
1/4 cup apple cider vinegar
2 tbsp chopped onion
2 cloves garlic, chopped
1/2 tsp dried whole oregano
Pinches of rosemary and thyme
1/2 tsp dry mustard powder
1/2 tsp paprika
1/2 of a roasted red bell pepper

Combine all ingredients in a blender container. Blend to mix thoroughly.

My Favorite Dressing
I use it often, as I no longer buy pre-made salad dressings.

Apple Cider Vinegar
High quality olive oil (I use Lucini from Italy)
Dijon mustard, organic
Raw honey
Fresh garlic, squeezed
Himalayan salt
Freshly ground black pepper
Fresh or dried dill (optional)

Whisk all together, pour on salad just before serving.

Spinach and Ginger (or Garlic) Ricotta
This light, low-carbohydrate breakfast or lunch dish combines two of my favorite ingredients - greens and fresh ginger or garlic. Organic baby spinach or other baby greens work great in this recipe. I love this for breakfast!!

1 cup organic spinach leaves
1 free ranged organic egg
1 egg white (or two eggs)
1 tsp fresh grated ginger root or garlic
Himalayan see salt and fresh pepper
1 tsp Italian or other seasoning mix (optional)
1 tbsp salsa (optional)

Tear up the spinach leaves and steam 3 minutes. Fold into the beaten eggs with the grated ginger or garlic add salt and pepper to taste. Add salsa and seasoning if desired. Cook on a non-stick pan sprayed with cooking spray, turning as needed until the eggs are set.

Warm Spinach Salad
1 red onion
Olive oil
2 cups sliced organic mushrooms
Sea salt
Fresh ground pepper
½ cup torn parsley
10 ounces spinach
Juice of 1 lemon
½ cup organic feta cheese

Cook onion in oil until golden, add mushrooms, cook until brown, and add salt. Off the heat, stir in parsley, spinach, and lemon juice. Season with salt and pepper, sprinkle with feta.

Cole Slaw
Great addition to a meal, or meal by itself.

1 cup shredded red cabbage
1 cup shredded green cabbage
½ carrot, shredded
¼ cup shredded white onion
1 tbsp cumin seeds
Juice from 1 lemon
1 tsp Himalayan sea salt
2 garlic cloves, minced
1 tsp ground cumin
1/3 cup olive oil
Drizzle of raw cider vinegar
1 medium tomato, diced (optional)

Mix all of the ingredients together in a large bowl, and serve.

Bell Pepper Slaw
Agave or Stevia to taste
Himalayan sea salt and freshly ground pepper to taste
½ cub apple cider vinegar
1 ½ tsp celery seeds
1 ½ tsp mustard seeds
6 bell peppers, all colors, cut into thin strips
2 stalk celery, finely chopped
4 scallions, chopped
½ head green cabbage, thinly sliced and roughly chopped
3 tbsp whole-grain Dijon mustard
½ cup Vegenaise (mayonnaise made from vegetables)

Wisk Agave and salt with vinegar. Add celery seeds, mustard seeds, pepper, bell peppers, celery, scallions and cabbage, toss. Refrigerate for at least an hour. Add mustard and Vegenaise and toss.

Organic Pizza
I make this pizza often, everybody likes it. My veggies change, depends on what I find in my fridge. Often I use only garlic, zucchini, and sun dried tomatoes in addition to cheese. Amazing taste.

Gluten-free pizza dough (Central Market has the best: 'Ancient Grain Pizza Crust')

Few gloves of garlic, sliced
Orange or red bell peppers, thinly sliced
Cherry tomatoes, halved
Zucchini, thinly sliced
Fresh mushrooms, thinly sliced
Spinach
Organic pizza sauce or tomato paste
1 1/4 c fresh lite mozzarella slices, organic from Central Market
1/2 c organic feta cheese, crumbled, from Central Market
Use organic vegetables.

Preheat oven to 400 degrees. Place pizza dough on baking stone, spread the pizza sauce, arrange the shredded mozzarella, veggies, feta over the top. Bake for 20-25 minutes.

Pizza Sauce
2 tbsp extra virgin olive oil
3 cloves garlic, minced
1 (6 oz) jar organic tomato paste
2/3 cup water
2 tbls red wine
5 drops of Stevia
1/2 te dried oregano
1/4 tsp dried basil
sea salt
pepper

Prep all the ingredients first and have them sitting ready to go. The recipe cooks fast, so this step is important.
In a medium saucepan, sauté garlic in oil until golden.
Add tomato paste, water, wine, Stevia, oregano, and basil.
Season with salt and pepper, to taste.
Simmer for 10 minutes over medium low heat. Remove from heat and spread over pizza dough.
Covers two medium pizzas or one large pizza.

Raw Spaghetti
3 pounds yellow summer squash

Pesto Sauce:
1 cup pine nuts

1 cup olive oil
½ large bunch fresh basil
½ cup chopped fresh parsley
3 garlic cloves
1 tbsp Himalayan sea salt

Thinly slice the yellow squash to create strands of "pasta". For the pesto sauce, put all the ingredients in a blender and blend until creamy. Toss the pesto sauce with the sliced squash pasta.

Ewa's Noodle Salad
Gluten-free noodles of your choice
Mushrooms
Swiss Chart (green)
Fresh oregano, 2 TBS
Fresh parsley, 3 TBS
Lemon, fresh squeeze + skin for zest
Fresh basil
Garlic, 8 gloves
Cayman pepper
Parmesan cheese

Cook noodles, sauté all other ingredients in olive oil, mix together with noodles, sprinkle with parmesan cheese and fresh basil. Yummy!!!

Pineapple & Cucumber salad by Kathy
Kathy likes to create her own recipes, here is one I like.

1 1/2 cup of pineapple diced
1 1/2 cup of cucumber peeled & diced
1/4 cup finely chopped red onion
1 tsp of finely chopped garlic
Red pepper flakes to taste
Himalayan sea salt to taste
Fresh ground black pepper to taste
Extra virgin olive oil - about 2-3 tablespoons
Juice of 1 lemon
Juice of 1 lime
Juice of small blood orange or 1/2 navel orange

1 tsp fresh parsley chopped fine (add more of less to your taste)
1 tsp of fresh mint chopped fine (add more or less to your taste)
Use small amount of zest from the lemon or lime to taste

Combine all ingredients in bowl. It's good to let this sit for at least 1/2 an hour before serving so the flavors come together. Great on fish, or over buckwheat and quinoa.

Beet and Arugula Salad

Beets are strong cancer fighters. Not many people like them; I love their flavor and think that everyone should find ways to eat them. Here are few.

1/2 lb arugula
1 small bunch beets without leaves (about 3 medium)
1 tbsp apple cider vinegar
1/4 cup olive oil

Peel beets and cut into 1/2-inch wedges. In a steamer set over boiling water, steam beets until tender, about 10 minutes, and transfer to a bowl. Discard course stems from arugula. Wash arugula well and dry. In a bowl whisk together vinegar and salt and pepper to taste and whisk in oil until emulsified. Pour half of vinaigrette over beets and toss well. To vinaigrette remaining in bowl add arugula and toss well. Arrange arugula and beets on 2 plates. Serves 2.

OR

Just boil whole beets for about 40 minutes or until a fork can slide through them. Then just drain, slice and drizzle olive oil over them. Sprinkle with sea salt and for added flavor and nutritional benefits, chop and toss some fresh green onion and organic cilantro over the top. Three or four large beets make a tasty meal, while one or two make a great side dish.

More Beets

3 medium beets
2 cloves garlic, pressed or chopped

2 tbsp fresh lemon juice
1 tbsp apple cider vinegar
3 tbsp extra virgin olive oil
Himalayan sea salt and black pepper to taste
10 fresh basil leaves, chopped

Cut beets into quarters and steam them, do not peel them.
Beets are cooked when you can easily insert a fork. Peel beets,
transfer to bowl and toss with remaining ingredients while they
are still hot.

Potato and Sweet Potato Torte
Layers of potatoes and sweet potatoes meld into an impressive
vegetable "cake" that forms a golden crust during baking. I
served it with free ranged turkey on Thanksgiving, everybody
liked it. Remember that even though potatoes are a whole food
they score high on both the glycemic index and glycemic load.
Eat them seldom and always choose organic red.

1 tbsp extra-virgin olive oil
2 large leeks, trimmed, washed and thinly sliced
1 tbsp chopped fresh thyme or 1 tsp dried thyme leaves
1/2 tsp Himalayan sea salt, or to taste
Freshly ground pepper to taste
1 pound yams or sweet potatoes (about 2 small), peeled and
cut into 1/8-inch-thick slices
1 pound red potatoes, peeled and cut into 1/8-inch-thick slices

Preheat to 450°F. Coat a 9 1/2-inch, deep-dish pie pan with
cooking spray. Line the bottom with parchment paper and
lightly coat with cooking spray.
Heat oil in a large nonstick skillet over medium-high heat. Add
leeks and thyme; cook, stirring often, until tender, about 5
minutes. (If necessary, add 1 to 2 tablespoons water to prevent
scorching.) Season with 1/8 teaspoon salt and pepper.
Sometimes I add organic mushrooms and fresh garlic.
Arrange half the sweet potato slices, slightly overlapping, in the
prepared pie pan and season with a little of the remaining salt
and pepper. Spread one-third of the leeks over the top. Arrange
half the potato slices over the leeks and season with salt and
pepper. Top with another third of the leeks. Layer the

remaining sweet potatoes, leeks and potatoes in the same manner. Cover the pan tightly with foil.
Bake the torte until the vegetables are tender, about 60 minutes. Run a knife around the edge of the torte to loosen it.

Raw Ketchup
An all raw organic version of one of my favorites sauces.

2 tomatoes chopped
¼ cup raw apple cider vinegar
¼ cup soaked sundried tomatoes
Dash of Agave or Stevia
Sea salt to taste

Blend all of ingredients and pour into a serving bowl.

Green Beans
I have made this recipe many times, great side dish or dish of its own if beans are placed on quinoa.

1 lb green beans
2 tsp fresh lemon juice
2 medium cloves garlic, chopped
3 tbsp extra vigin olive oil
Himalayan sea salt and pepper to taste
3 tbsp goat or feta cheese
2 tbsp sliced almonds
4-5 drops Bragg Liquid Aminos
1 tbsp sliced sun dried tomatoes
2 tbsp roasted red bell peppers
1 tbsp chopped fresh basil

Chop garlic.
Fill the bottom of a steamer pot with 2 inches of water. While steam is building up in steamer, cut ends off green beans, steam for 5 minutes. A fork should pierce through them easily when they are done.
Transfer to a bowl. For more flavor, toss green beans with the remaining ingredients while they are still hot.

Green Beans, Red Potatoes, Cherry Tomatoes Salad

Every time I make it I get compliments, so make it for your friends too.

2 lbs. organic baby red potatoes, halved
Sea salt
1 lb. Green beans, trimmed and cut in half
3 Tbs. Apple cider vinegar
1 Tbs. whole-grain Dijon mustard
3/4 cup extra-virgin olive oil
1 medium shallot, finely diced (about 3 Tbs.)
1 Tbs. chopped fresh thyme
Freshly ground black pepper
2 Tbs. capers, rinsed and drained
1 pint cherry tomatoes, halved
3/4 cup pitted Niçoise or Kalamata olives, chopped

Boil potatoes, steam green beans, make sure they are not too soft. Drain well and cool under running water.

In a blender blend the vinegar with the mustard. With the machine still running, add the oil in a slow, steady stream so the mixture comes together into a thick emulsion. Add the shallot, thyme, salt, and pepper, and purée until incorporated. Taste and season the dressing with more salt and pepper if needed. Add 1 or 2 Tbs. water if needed to thin the dressing to a pourable consistency.
Transfer the potatoes, beans and tomatoes to a large mixing bowl and toss well with the vinaigrette. Taste and season with salt and pepper if needed and transfer to a large platter.
Sprinkle with the remaining 1 tsp. thyme and capers and serve.

Greek Salad

There are many variations of Greek Salad, this is the healthiest I found. Use organic ingredients.

1/2 cucumber diced
1/4 red bell pepper diced
1/4 orange pepper diced
1/4 yellow pepper diced
1/4 green pepper diced
1 cup cherry tomatoes

2 fresh lemons squeezed
2 Tablespoons olive oil
1 tsp oregano

Wash and dice all vegetables than put them in a large bowl. Combine lemon juice, olive oil, and oregano and pour over salad.

Carrots and Broccoli with Ume Dill Dressing
2 cups water
1 pinch sea salt
2 cups organic carrot chunks
2 cups organic broccoli

Dressing: 1/4 cup olive oil, 2 TBL apple cider vinegar, pinch sea salt, fresh dill

1. Bring water and salt to a boil. Quickly blanch carrots and remove from the water. Re-boil the water and quickly blanch the broccoli and remove. Each should be bright and crunchy. Let cool separately.
2. When cool, arrange carrots and broccoli in a beautiful clear bowl.
3. Mix the dressing ingredients and toss with veggies. Let set 5-10 minutes so the dressing can marinade the vegetables.

Lemon Broccoli
2 minced garlic cloves
2 or 3 strips lemon zest
3 tablespoons olive oil
Broccoli florets
1 sliced carrot
Chopped tomato (optional)

Heat garlic with lemon zest and olive oil in a skillet over medium, 3 minutes. Meanwhile steam 1 head broccoli florets and carrot. Toss with the lemon oil, squeeze lemon juice, and salt and pepper. Add tomato.

Tabouli Salad with Quinoa

Tabouli, a delicious Middle Eastern salad, was always one of my favorite foods. Here is a healthy version.

1 cup organic quinoa
1 1/2 tsp Himalayan salt
1/4 cup lemon or lime juice
2 tbsp olive oil, extra virgin
4 tbsp green onions
1 cup parsley
1 1/2 cup cilantro
1/2 cup fresh mint
4 tomatoes

Wash 1/2 cup quinoa seeds, add 1 cup water, salt, and tsp olive oil. Bring it to boil than simmer until quinoa is ready. ½ cub of raw quinoa will change to 1 cup once is cooked. Chap all vegetables, mix with quinoa, lemon juice, olive oil, and salt to taste. Place in fridge for at least two hours before eating.

Cauliflower Tabouli

1 head cauliflower
2 diced plum tomatoes
½ cup fresh lemon juice
3 tablespoons olive oil
2 tablespoons Bragg Liquid Aminos (healthy version of soy sauce)
2 scallions
Bunch parsley
2 tablespoons chopped mint
Sea salt
Fresh ground pepper

Grate cauliflower into grain-size pieces with a box grater. Toss with diced tomatoes, lemon juice, olive oil, soy sauce, scallions, parsley, and mint. Add salt and pepper to taste.

Honey Glazed Carrots

1 ¼ pounds organic carrots, peeled
1 tablespoon raw butter
1 ½ tablespoon raw honey

1 tablespoon fresh lemon juice

Stem carrots for 4 to 8 minutes or until tender, transfer to a bowl. In a skillet melt the butter with the honey and lemon juice, stirring until the mixture is smooth, add the carrots. Cook the mixture over.low heat, stirring, for 1 to 2 minutes, or until carrots are glazed evenly, season with sea salt and fresh pepper.

Steamed Kale
Kale is not the best tasting vegetable; however, with the right recipe it can be very delicious. Besides we must include it in our diet for the strong health benefits. I learned to LOVE IT!

1 lb kale
1 tsp quality extra-virgin olive oil
2 cloves garlic, minced
1/2 cup water
1 tsp cider vinegar
Sea salt and pepper to taste

Wash the kale well by submerging it in clean water a couple of times. Use a sharp knife to cut out the ribs of the kale and coarsely chop the leaves. In a large skillet with a lid, heat the oil. Sauté the garlic until it just begins to turn golden. Add the kale and the water. Stir briefly and cover. Cook on medium until the kale is tender but still bright green. Sprinkle with vinegar, season to taste and serve.

Patti's Kale
Patti made it for me and I loved it.

1 Bunch of Organic Kale
2 chopped Garlic cloves or 2 chopped Shallots
2 - 3 tablespoons spoons of Olive oil in pan
Sun-dried Tomatoes 1/4 cup chopped
1/4 cup White Wine (inexpensive chardonnay for example)
Toasted Almond Slivers - 3- 4 Tablespoons (optional)

Toast almond slivers before you begin cooking the kale in a small frying pan without oil.

Wash the Kale and cut out the large stems. Steam it for 3 -5 minutes to take out the bitterness.

Sauté the garlic or shallots until slightly brown then add the Sun-dried tomatoes and continue to sauté for another 1 -2 minutes... now add the kale and sauté for about 2 - 3 minutes drizzling it with about 1/4 cup of white wine at the end. (The pan should be hot for this part as the alcohol will cook off leaving only a lovely flavor on the kale.) Sprinkle with toasted almonds and serve.

Salmon with Honey-Mustard Sauce

I like wild salmon; this is the recipe I use a lot.

¼ cup Dijon mustard
2 tablespoons raw honey
2 tablespoons prepared horseradish, drained
2 tablespoons finely chopped fresh mint leaves
Sea salt and freshly ground black pepper
2 pound wild fresh salmon, skin on
2 tablespoons olive oil

Whisk together the mustard, honey, horseradish, mint, salt and pepper in a small bowl. Let sit for at least 15 minutes before using.

Brush the salmon with the oil and season with salt and pepper. Bake it for 10-12 minutes in 450 degrees. Drizzle salmon with mustard sauce and serve.

Mustard Dill Sauce

I use this with Salmon.

4 oz silken tofu
1 TBS prepared mustard such as Dijon
4 TBS fresh dill chopped
1 TBS honey
2 TBS fresh lemon juice
1/2 cup water
1/4 tsp sea salt
1/4 tsp white pepper
2 TBS extra virgin olive oil

Place all sauce ingredients, except olive oil, in a blender and begin to blend on high speed for about one minute. While blender is running, drizzle olive oil in a little at a time. Set aside. Steam asparagus until is tender, about 3-5 minutes, depending on thickness. Remove from steamer, toss with 1 TBS lemon juice, 1 TBS olive oil, salt and pepper.

Rub salmon with 1 TBS lemon juice and season with a little salt and pepper. Place salmon in the same steamer basket and steam until pink inside, about 3-4 minutes. Place salmon on a plate and pour desired amount of sauce over it and the asparagus.

Seafood with Asparagus

I like this recipe because includes variety of seafood and vegetables.

1 medium onion, cut in half and sliced medium thick
1 TBS chicken or vegetable broth
1 TBS minced fresh ginger
3 medium cloves garlic, chopped
2 cups fresh sliced shiitake mushrooms
1 bunch thin asparagus, cut in 2" lengths (discard bottom fourth)
¼ cup fresh lemon juice
2 TBS tamari or Bragg Liquid Aminos
pinch red pepper flakes
3/4 lb cod fillet cut into 1 inch pieces
8 large scallops
8 large shrimp, peeled and deveined
1 cup cherry tomatoes cut in quarters
¼ cup chopped fresh cilantro
Sea salt and fresh pepper to taste

Slice onion and chop garlic. Heat 1 TBS broth in a stainless steel wok or 12 inch skillet. Add onion in broth over medium high heat for 2 minutes, stirring constantly. Add ginger, garlic, and mushrooms. Continue to stir-fry for another 3 minutes, stirring constantly. Steam asparagus, make sure is still half hard.

Add lemon juice, Bragg, red pepper flakes, cod, scallops, shrimp and asparagus and stir to mix well. Cover and simmer for just about 5 minutes stirring occasionally on medium heat. Toss in tomatoes, cilantro, salt and pepper.

Garlic-Basil Shrimp

This recipe is easy and delicious and takes short time to cook.

2 tbsp olive oil
1 ¼ lb large shrimp, peeled and deveined
3 garlic cloves, minced
1/8 tsp crushed red pepper flakes
¾ cup dry white wine
1 ½ cups organic grape tomatoes, halved
¼ cup finely chopped fresh basil
Sea salt and freshly ground pepper to taste

Heat the oil in a large heavy skillet over medium-high heat until hot but not smoking, then add shrimp and cook, turning over once, until just cooked through, about 2 minutes. Transfer with a slotted spoon to a large bowl.
Add garlic and red pepper flakes to the remaining oil and cook until fragrant, about 30 seconds. Add the wine and cook over high heat, stirring occasionally, for 3 minutes. Stir in tomatoes and basil and season the sauce with salt and pepper.

Return the shrimp to the pan and cook just until heated.

Sautéed Chicken Breast

1 medium onion cut in half and sliced medium thick
5 medium cloves garlic, pressed
2 organic boneless, skinless chicken breasts, cut into 1-inch pieces
3 TBS Dijon mustard
1 TBS + ½ cup chicken broth
2 tsp honey
1 TBS chopped fresh tarragon (or 1 tsp dried tarragon)
2 TBS chopped fresh parsley (or 2 tsp dried parsley)
Sea salt and fresh pepper to taste

Slice onion and press. Heat 1 TBS broth in a 10-12 inch stainless steel skillet. Sautè onion in broth over medium heat for 2 minutes. While onions are sautéing, cut chicken into pieces. Add chicken pieces and continue to sauté for another 3 minutes, stirring frequently to seal chicken on all sides. Add garlic and continue to sauté for another minute.

Add mustard, ½ cup broth, and honey. Mix thoroughly and simmer uncovered for about 7-8 minutes on medium-high heat stirring occasionally to cook chicken evenly. This will also reduce sauce. While chicken is cooking, chop herbs and add at end with salt and pepper to taste.

Gazpacho Soup
This is my favorite summer soup.

1 hothouse cucumber, halved and seeded, but not peeled
1 organic red bell pepper, cored and seeded
1 organic green bell pepper, cored and seeded
4 organic plum tomatoes, peeled and seeded
1 red onion
3 garlic cloves, finely minced
3 cups organic tomato juice
1/4 cup white wine vinegar
1/4 cup organic olive oil
1/2 tablespoon Himalayan sea salt
1 teaspoons freshly ground black pepper
Juice of 1 lime
Handful of chopped cilantro
Avocado for garnish (optional)

Roughly chop into 1 inch cubes, cucumbers, bell peppers, tomatoes, and red onion. Place each vegetable separately into a food processor fitted with a steel blade and pulse until it is coarsely chopped. It is important to NOT overprocess! After each vegetable is processed, combine them in a large bowl and add the garlic, tomato juice, vinegar, olive oil, lime juice, salt, and pepper. Mix well and chill before serving. The longer gazpacho sits, the more the flavors develop. Garnish with cilantro and/or avocado before serving.

Sandwich

The combination of bread and vegetables that typically comprises the sandwich can be perfectly balanced and healthy. Sandwiches used to be serious part of my diet, they still are; however, I make them differently. Here are two good recipes.

First:
Ezekiel bread
Chopped red onions
Garlic
Parsley
Basil
Tomatoes
Avocado
Sea salt
Spread avocado on bread, combine all ingredients and spread on top of avocado.

Second:
Spread avocado on Ezekiel bread, on top place cucumber slices, then radish slices, sea salt and black pepper, finally alfala sprouts.

Smoked Salmon Scramble

Smoked wiled salmon
Ezekiel bread
1 tablespoon coconut oil
2 free ranged eggs
2 tablespoons chives
Sea salt
Freshly grounded pepper

Scramble over medium heat eggs with chopped chives, add two tablespoons organic cottage cheese, cheese is optional. Add salt and pepper. Serve on toasted bread with smoked salmon.

Olive Paste

1 13-ounce jar pitted raw olives (preferably Nature's First Law Italian)

Puree the olives in a blender, adding enough juice from the olive jar to achive desired thickness. Spread on Ezekiel bread for hors d'oeuvres.

Glow Nectar
This juice is secret to good health and abundant energy.

2 cucumbers
Celery
Broccoli Stalks
Sweet pea sprouts, sunflower sprouts, or both
Kale
Throw everything into the juicer or blender.

Buckwheat (Kasha) – refer to March 9

Salsa & Guacamole – refer to May 3

References and Sources:

February 3: From article by Mike Adams
in http://www.naturalnews.com,
February 6: "Cancer Free" book by Bill Henderson, "Definitive
Guide to Cancer" book by Lisa Alschuler and Karolyn Gazella;
for Amazon Herbs go to
Herbswin.amazonherb.net, http://drbenkim.com/cancer-
prevention-antioxidants.htm,
February 11: "Cancer Free" book by Bill Henderson
February 13: Journal of Clinical Oncology, September
2005, http://www.healthyeatingadvisor.com/healthy-food.html,
February 21: "Alternatives in Cancer Therapy" book by Ross
Perlton and Lee Overholsten, Paul S Fitzgerald -
EzineArticles.com, "The Cure: Heal your body, save your
life" book by Timothy Brantley, "The Live Food Factor, The
Comprehesive Guide to the Ultimate Diet for Body and Mind,
Spirit& Planet" by Susan Schenck
February 22:' The China Study' book by Dr. T. Colin Campbell
http://products.mercola.com/produce/free-range-ostrich/
February 23: ""Healing The Gerson Way, Defeating Cancer and
Other Chronic Diseases" book by Charlotte Gerson with Beata
Bishop; http://www.ralphmoss.com/coff.html, http://curezone.
com/art/read.asp?ID=28&db=5&C0=818, http://www.modern
manna.org/coffee_enema.asp,
February 25: Navarro Medical Clinic, DR. Efren Navarro,
Philippines
February
26: www.ewg.org, http://www.naturalnews.com/026802_probi
otic_probiotics_disease.html, http://www.naturalnews.com/027
518_probiotics_food_allergies.html,
March 1: Books by Eckhart Tolle
March 2: http://organizedhome.com/clean-house/pantry-
recipes-homemade-cleaning-
products, http://www.doityourself.com/stry/makecleansupply,
http://www.aroma-essence.com/house-
cleaning.html, http://hubpages.com/hub/Top-10-Essential-Oils-
for-House-Cleaning,
http://www.whfoods.com/genpage.php?pfriendly=1&tname=ge
orge&dbid=99
March 3: "Back To The House Of Health" book by Shelley Young,
, "Easy ways to balance an Acidic Diet", article written by Dr.
Phil Domenico, http://www.naturallydirect.net/alkaline-cancer-

natural-healing.htm, http://www.thewolfeclinic.com/phbalancearticle.html, http://www.antiagingresearch.com/ph_balance_rx.shtml,
March 4: http://www.ionizers.org/water.html, http://hydrogenfriends.com/hydrogen-friends-university/special-reports/dont-buy-an-ionizer, http://www.naturalnews.com/026605_fluoride_fluorides_detox.html, http://www.nofluoride.com/, http://www.liquidzeoliteplus.com/flouride_dangers.html,
March 7: http://drbenkim.com/articles-vitamins.html, http://www.nutriteam.com/natural.htm, http://library.thinkquest.org/26813/importance.htm,
March 9: http://www.naturalnews.com/025985_wheat_buckwheat_bacteria.html, http://hsibaltimore.com/2003/06/18/the-health-benefits-of-buckwheat, about quinoa www.bodyenclogy.com,
March 11: Bentonite calcium: http://www.naturalnews.com/027487_clay_bentonite_calcium.html, http://www.aboutclay.com/info/how_clay_works.htm,
Mercury: http://articles.mercola.com/sites/articles/archive/2002/08/14/mercury-part-six.aspx, http://www.noharm.org/all_regions/issues/toxins/mercury/,
March 16: Book 'Health Begins in The Colon' by Dr. Group, chart: http://www.hsu.com/food_combining_simplified.htm,
March 26: http://www.naturalnews.com/027123_cancer_Tamoxifen_brst_cancer.html, http://www.fhcrc.org/about/ne/news/2009/08/25/tamoxifen.html,
March 27: http://www.bodybasics.vpweb.com/,
March 30: Rudy Silva, nutritionist and writer of natural remedies, www.constipationcured.info and www.stop-constipation.com
April 1: "Cancer-Free: Your Guide to Gentle, Non-Toxic Healing" book by Bill Henderson
April 7: http://www.pickthebrain.com/blog/10-ways-to-instantly-build-self-confidence/,
April 8: http://www.alternativesmagazine.com/28/lipton.html,
April 9: http://drbenkim.com/organ-systems.htm,
April 11:
Telomeres: http://users.rcn.com/jkimball.ma.ultranet/BiologyPages/T/Telomeres.html,

Resveratrol: Science Daily August 3 2009, The FASEB Journal August 2009

Beta Glucan: www.bestbetaglucan.com

April 13: Walnuts: http://www.aacr.org/home/public--media/aacr-press-releases.aspx?d=1321, http://www.ncbi.nlm.nih.gov/pubmed/15037535, http://www.naturalnews.com/026115_walnuts_health_cancer.html,

Pineapple: http://www.naturalnews.com/026064.html, http://www.elements4health.com/pineapple.html,

April 14: Book by Timothy Brantley "The Cure: Heal your body, save your life", http://www.associatedcontent.com/article/1185306/why_is_ezekiel_bread_healthy.html?cat=22, http://www.wheat-free.org/wheat-free-flour.html. http://articles.mercola.com/sites/articles/archive/2010/08/25/why-has-this-lifesustaining-essential-nutrient-been-vilified-by-doctors.aspx,

April 22: http://www.stress.org/newsletterview-WHY-DO-HAPPY-PEOPLE-OPTIMISTS-LIVE-LONGER--144.htm,

May 1: "Cancer – 50 Essential Things To Do" book by Greg Anderson

May 3: http://www.naturalnews.com/026246_guacamole_cilantro_salt.html,

May 6: 'Asparagus for cancer' printed in Cancer News Journal, December 1979,

Mushrooms: http://www.naturalnews.com/026495_cancer_mushrooms_breast_cancer.html,

Papaya: http://www.naturalnews.com/025846_papaya_health_food.html, http://www.whfoods.com/genpage.php?tname=food spice&dbid=47,

May 12: http://ezinearticles.com/?Breast-Cancer-Causes---5-Reasons-Why-You-Have-Breast-Cancer&id=2113624, http://articles.mercola.com/sites/articles/archive/2009/05/19/Can-Wearing-Your-Bra-Cause-Cancer.aspx, http://www.selfstudycenter.org/dressedtokill.htm, http://www.relfe.com/underwire_bras_dangers.html, http://www.thecellphonechipstore.com

MASY 14: Warburg O. On the origin of cancer cells. Science 1956 Feb;123:309-14. http://articles.mercola.com/sites/articles/archive/2010/08/27/warning--fructose-feeds-cancer-cells.aspx,

May

16: http://www.iowasource.com/health/2009_04_b12.html, http://www.ajcn.org/cgi/content/abstract/89/2/693S, http://articles.mercola.com/sites/articles/archive/2009/05/19/Warning-Potentially-Life-Threatening-Vitamin-Deficiency-Affects-25-Percent-of-Adults.aspx,

May

17: http://www.naturalteacher.com/NTArticleDangerousSkinCareIngredients.html, Dr. Mercola

from www.mercolahealthyskin.com/skincare-offer.aspx,

May 24: "Timpless Secrets of Health & Rejuvenation" book by Andreas Morik, www.jimhumble.biz

June 5: Dr. Ray

Strand, http://www.naturalnews.com/026399_cancer_CoQ10_health.html, http://www.talkmydisease.com/topic653.html,

June 9: Mike Adams, the Health Ranger; Natural News; Dr. Ariel Policano, naturopathic physician with a special focus on women's health

June

13: http://articles.mercola.com/sites/articles/archive/2009/04/28/Primary-Principles-of-Exercise-Aerobic-Interval-Strength-Core.aspx,

June 16 & 17: book written by Tommy Newberry, "The 4:8 Principle"

June

20: http://www.breastthermography.com/breast_thermography_mf.htm, http://www.infiniteunknown.net/2009/12/03/mammograms-cause-breast-cancer-groundbreaking-new-research-declares/,

June 22: http://www.nutritional-supplement-educational-centre.com/amino-acid-benefits.html, http://ezinearticles.com/?amino-acid---benefits-and-its-functions&id=338913,

July 1: Dr. Maret Traber, "Alternatives in Cancer Therapy" book by Ross Perlton and Lee Overholsten

July

5: http://www.fourwinds10.com/siterun_data/health/food/news.php?q=1257442576, www.centerforfoodsafety.org, www.healthiereating.org, http://www.nongmoshoppingguide.com/SG/Home/index.cfm, http://www.sustainabletable.org/issues/additives/,

July

7: http://life.gaiam.com/gaiam/p/10WaystoDetoxifyYourBody.h

tml, http://www.naturalnews.com/026586_toxins_detox_water. html, http://themastercleanserecipe.org/, http://mastercleanse secrets.com/index.php,

July
8: http://www.naturalnews.com/026559_coffee_health_chemic als.html, http://www.wereyouwondering.com/what-role-does-the-liver-play-in-the-human-body/,

July
10: http://articles.mercola.com/sites/articles/archive/2004/06/ 23/antioxidants-free-radicals.aspx,

July
11: http://altmedicine.about.com/od/popularhealthdiets/a/Raw _Food.htm, http://www.nzherald.co.nz/diabetes/news/article.cf m?c_id=174&objectid=10117603, http://www.naturalnews.co m/026238.html,

July
18: http://articles.mercola.com/sites/articles/archive/2009/07/ 09/Changing-Your-Beliefs-About-Health-and-Illness.aspx, rom interview with Dr. Pizzarno by Mike Adams

July 22: from article by Ellie Krieger for Heathy Living, Book by Timothy Brantley "The Cure: Heal your body, save your life"

July 23: "Natural Health, Natural Medicine" book by Andrew Weil, http://www.herbwisdom.com, http://www.diffen.com/diff erence/Saturated_Fats_vs_Unsaturated_Fats, http://www.west onaprice.org,

August 2: Book by Mary-Ann Shearer "Perfect Health: The Natural Ways"

August 3: Book by Ray Strand "Healthy for Life"

August 8: http://naturalhealthcenter.mercola.com

August
21: http://www.naturalnews.com/026847_honey_raw_honey_f ood.html, http://www.westonaprice.org/Fermented-Honey.html

August
31: www.themiraclemineralsupplement.com, www.jimhumble.b iz

September 7 and 11: Book 'Health Begins in The Colon' by Dr. Group, http://www.bodybasics.vpweb.com/,

September
17: http://www.naturalnews.com/027032_beets_cancer_tumor s.html, http://www.betterbe.ca/Documents/Ferenczi1959eng.p df,

September
19: http://www.naturalnews.com/027345_Vitamin_D_sun_exp

osure_blood.html, http://whfoods.org/genpage.php?tname=nutrient&dbid=110, http://www.vitamindcouncil.org/, http://articles.mercola.com/sites/articles/archive/2009/10/10/Vitamin-D-Experts-Reveal-the-Truth.aspx, http://www.urmc.rochester.edu/news/story/index.cfm?id=2647,

September 26: Book by Timothy Brantley "The Cure: Heal your body, save your life"

http://www.wehealny.org/healthinfo/dietaryfiber/index.html#Twenty for The Top Twenty Fiber Foods

September 27:

http://www.drmercola.com, http://www.betaglucan.org, http://www.newhope.com/nutritionsciencenews/NSN_backs/Jan_01/betaglucan.cfm,

www.ingramcontent.com/pod-product-compliance
Lightning Source LLC
Chambersburg PA
CBHW072043280526
45788CB00006B/2162